TO HEALTH STEP BY STEP

TERRY ABEL

DEDICATION

*I dedicate this book to my beautiful and wonderful God.
The Divine Presence who guides me and supports me every step of the way.
Without your intervention in my daily affairs, I would not be where I am.
THANK YOU!
And, of course, to my lovely parents who gave me the opportunity to experience life!
To Rick, your transition guided me to a healthier path. See you in our next adventure!
And to my gorgeous Tuxedo who left the day after Thanksgiving. I love you sweetheart!*

TERRY ABEL

CONTENTS

TERRY ABEL

ACKNOWLEDGEMENTS

A very special thank you to **Dr. Howard Loomis Jr.** from *Loomis Food Enzyme Institute* who was one of the very first people to impact my life. I am forever grateful for your immense generosity and wealth of information you have shared with humanity. You have steered me toward a great path to health. I have so much to learn from you!!!

And to **Dr. Ritamarie Loscalzo** who has been the second most important figure in my journey to health. You have catapulted me to the next level. I continually learn from you.

Thank you both for being in my experience.

And to my other teachers who have enriched my life:

Dr. Philip Fritchey
Dr. Thomas Anstett
Dr. Elaine Newkirk
Dr. Marcus Shumway

AUTHOR'S NOTE

The majority of individuals, when encountered with the word "health" automatically relate it to food and exercise; this is not totally true. My definition of health is finding a balance among all areas of life: body, mind, emotions, and spirit. It does not mean following a diet until you reach your desired goal and then reverting to your previous habits, or going overboard with exercise and then letting it go because you have also reached a target. Health means incorporating changes that YOU KNOW you will maintain for the rest of your life; small changes that will have an impact in your quality of life as you grow in years. The key words here are FOR THE REST OF YOUR LIFE until it becomes a habit.

But how? How can you achieve the right life style for you? How can you make sense of all the information that is out there? How can you implement it in your life?

This book offers you an easy step-by-step program to help you implement small to big changes one at a time and it helps you make sense of all those healthful superfoods. There is no order to follow. Choose one tip randomly and implement it, and then another, and another, and another; you will find yourself moving effortlessly through the health path. One day you will notice what a different life style you have accomplished without even feeling the change, and the PAY-OFF is huge: you have more energy; you definitely enjoy a better quality of sleep; you stop experiencing that afternoon slump. When you implement these tips, you accomplish **pain-free energetic living** and you literally have more LIFE.

We have been trained to believe in averages and scales. When someone comes up with these specific amounts of what everyone should eat or drink, I ask them:

Is a 5' (1.52 m) woman weighing 110 lbs (50 kg) the same as a 7' (2. 1 m) man weighing 180 lbs (82 kg)?
THERE IS NO AVERAGE PERSON! We are all unique and have different physiques, different genes, and different habits so it does not make sense to have the same parameters and standards for everyone!

<u>I cannot emphasize enough what an incredible feeling it is to live pain-free at 60 years young. It is a true gift I have given myself through love and dedication and you can too.</u>

It is my strong desire to help as many individuals as possible. I sincerely hope this book helps you reach a healthier life style. It is not easy to give up many of our not-so-healthy habits. Throughout my path toward health I have learned many things, AND I am sure of one thing: **IF YOU WANT TO LIVE A HEALTHY LIFE**, there is no choice: **YOU HAVE TO PAY THE PRICE** by changing those habits. I tried many diets and exercise plans and I was *extremely successful* at reaching my weight goals, many weight goals throughout my 20's, 30's, and part of my 40's; and I ended up gaining even more because I never viewed it as a life-long commitment. My best advise to you is: DO NOT start something you are not willing to do for the rest of your life.

As I said before, the key lies in making small changes which will become life-long habits which will yield a longer, healthier, and more energetic life! **Your body is a beautiful and intelligent machine; DON'T TREAT IT VIOLENTLY**. If you listen to it, it will heal itself in time with patience and care. You are in control of your own body and habits. Don't let anyone or any thing stir you differently! **A doughnut cannot have and does not have any hidden dark power over you.** Use reverse psychology; imagine the doughnut as the worst enemy on Earth with an implacable desire to kill you! And then go on to another bad food.

BE AWARE OF YOUR BODY'S MESSAGES! If you pay attention to how you feel, your body will let you know when something is not right.

We all have two ages: the biological and the physical. ***Aim for a younger biological age!*** As someone said before: At the end: **YOU ARE THE CEO OF YOUR OWN HEALTH!!**

<u>DISCLAIMER: If you are breast-feeding, pregnant or have any ailment or disease, please check with your doctor before you make any changes to your lifestyle or diet. The information given here is solely intended for educational purposes and it is not intended to diagnose, treat, cure, or prevent disease nor to replace a doctor's advice.</u>

SO.......... **TO YOUR HEALTH!!!**

Check the Glossary at the end!!

LET'S START!!!!

TIP #1:

As you wake up, opening your eyes for the first time that day, stretch your body. Stretch your legs, stretch your arms, stretch your feet, stretch your hands, stretch your fingers. Watch Nature: Almost every animal upon awakening stretches its body, why won't we?

TIP #2:

Hug yourself and while you are doing so, tell yourself: "Wonderful Me!" "Wonderful Me!" "Wonderful Me!" Love yourself just the way you are right now, and miracles will ensue!

TIP #3:

Drink 8 to 16 ounces of pure WATER (1/4 to 1/2 litre appx), upon awakening. Have it ready by your nightstand so you remember to do this first thing in the morning. It will not only help your bowel movements, but also hydrate your body and your heart. See TIPS #4, #200, and #377.

TIP #4:

If you are not used to drinking water, add slices of FRESH lemon, lime, grapefruit, cucumber, mint, orange, etc. until you get used to drinking water. And then just transition to plain water. See TIPS #3 and #**200**.

TIP #5:

If you are used to drinking any beverage with white or brown sugar, replace the sugar with green stevia (white has already been processed), lucuma powder, organic dates, erythritol, xylitol (some individuals may experience diarrhea with this one), Jerusalem artichoke, raw honey or maple syrup. You can also use these substitutes (1:1 ratio) for baking or cooking. Please no pink, yellow, or blue packets; besides being chemically treated, they are also linked to many diseases. See TIP #35.

TIP #6:

Dry brush your skin in a circular pattern before taking a shower. Use a brush with natural bristles. Start with your feet and legs in an upward and circular motion always brushing toward your heart. Continue with your torso and then your arms, always toward the heart. It is a bit uncomfortable at the beginning, do not discourage; be gentle with yourself and, in time, you will be able to brush more vigorously. The biggest organ of your body is the skin and it is one of the organs of elimination. We need to clean it; we need to get rid of all the layers of dead cells we have built up. This will also improve your circulation and will allow your skin to breathe better.

TIP #7:

Have you heard of oil pulling? It is an ancient technique used to pull out "garbage" from your body. Before you get into the shower, take a mouthful of sesame seed oil (organic) and swish it in your mouth while you take a shower. DO NOT SWALLOW! Do this for a couple minutes while you shower. The mouth is one of the places where we accumulate more bacteria. Make sure you DO NOT dispose of the oil through your drain; it will clog it. Finish with your regular mouthwash.

TIP #8:

Switch your toothpaste and mouthwash to non-fluoridated brands. See TIPS #60, #82, and #202.

TIP #9:

Now let's get some energy going!..........Take a deep and continuous breath in through the nose (counting up to 20 very, very, very slowly), and exhale out through the mouth. (counting to twenty.........very.......very......slowly.) Make sure you do not use your chest to breathe; your chest should not move. Inflate your stomach, use that diaphragm!! Your belly should inflate when you inhale and deflate as you exhale. Watch how babies breathe! Do 10 to 20 repetitions before you get out of bed. Oxygen: precious element, cannot live without it!

TIP #10:

Mix 1 teaspoon of 100% organic raw apple cider vinegar with the mother with 1/4 to 1/2 glass of pure water.   Make sure you shake the bottle vigorously to mix it well. Apple cider vinegar has many properties: it is antibacterial and anti-fungal. It will soothe your sore throat, help with acne, and it is a digestive soother, among other things. I only use it when I have a sore throat.

TIP #11:

Take 1/2 teaspoon of royal jelly in the morning. It has many properties: great anti-tumor, antioxidant, antimicrobial, anti-inflammatory, disinfectant, energizes, to name a few. Take it as often as possible. It is a well-rounded food. I rotate royal jelly with bee pollen. See TIP#71.

TIP #12:

Green juice for life. There are many recipes out there. By the way, a green juice means just that: NO fruit, no dairy, ALL greens. I have chosen to start my day with the following juice:
1 cucumber
3 stalks of celery
3/4 cup of green beans
All through a slow-auger juicer.
Then I add:
1/8 tsp of cinnamon
1/8 tsp of turmeric
1/8 tsp of cardamom.
I use a low-speed juicer, and not a blender. These ingredients balance blood sugar and fight inflammation. This I do once or twice a week on average. See TIPS #30 and #203.

TIP #13:

Exercise to improve memory and brain power. Stand up straight with your feet shoulder width apart. Take your left hand and grab your right ear lobe and then take the right hand and grab the left ear lobe. Push your tongue toward the upper palate. Next, start squatting. Inhale as you go down and exhale as you come up. The National Center on

Health, Physical Activity, and Disability (NCHPAD) is using this exercise to improve the learning ability and focus for autistic children.

TIP #14:

Drink a smoothie as part of your breakfast. I use a blender to prepare it. The key to a smoothie is 2/3 leafy greens to 1/3 fruit. I have about 24 to 32 ounces of it 5 to 6 times a week. I did not start this way, I built up a little at a time. Again, the key is to be gentle with oneself. Start by using leafy lettuces such as romaine, butter, red-leaf, etc.; never iceberg. Add spinach too and lots of water with ice. Then build up. See TIP #100.

TIP #15:

No time for breakfast? Have an organic sliced apple - skin included - with a dozen of some sort of unsalted nuts, nut yoghurt, or nut butter, preferably organic: almonds, pecans, walnuts, cashews, etc. If you are short on time, you can take this and eat it on your way to work.

TIP #16:

Here are some ideas for healthful snacks: Pico de gallo, zucchini hummus, home-made salsas with veggies, hummus, soaked chia with apples and shredded unsweetened coconut, almond milk, cashew yogurt, organic raw nuts, raw organic celery, raw organic radishes, raw organic tomatoes, etc. Raw organic veggies in general. If you snack on meats and cheese, let them be organic and pasture-raised. See TIP #304.

TIP #17:

It is important to keep your eyes hydrated. I put 2 drops in each eye twice a day. Choose a brand that has individual applications because they do not have preservatives. In general, if drops are in a bottle, they have preservatives. See TIP #18.

TIP #18:

Just as we protect our skin from the sun, so should we protect our eyes. That is why it is important to use sunglasses; even babies should use sunglasses. Your eyesight will stay healthier longer. See TIP #17.

TIP #19:

Brush your hair, including the scalp, at least, 10 minutes every day. This will help circulation, luster, and growth. Use a brush with natural bristles.

TIP #20:

Try to eat organic if your budget allows it. If you are unable to do so, try to ALWAYS buy these following produce ORGANIC; by doing so, you are reducing about 50% of pesticides from your diet. The list is known as "The Dirty Dozen" and it might vary every year. The Environmental Working Group has more information. See TIPS #21, #76, #225, #241 and #306:

Apples
Celery
Cherries
Cucumbers

Grapes
Hot peppers
Nectarines
Peaches
Pears
Potatoes
Spinach
Strawberries
Sweet bell peppers
Tomatoes

This year the has expanded their list to add:
Leafy greens (especially kale and collards)
Summer squash (USA grown)

TIP #21:

Their is a list from the Environmental Working Group called
"The Clean 15". These produce do not need to be organic.
See TIPS #20, #76, #225, **#241** and #306:

Asparagus
Avocado
Cabbage
Cantaloupe
Sweet corn
Eggplant
Grapefruit
Kiwi
Mango
Mushrooms
Onion
Papaya
Pineapple
Sweet peas
Sweet potato

TIP #22:

When you are taking a shower, using soap, massage along the inner part of your shin using your thumb. Start at your ankle and move toward the knee. Do this 10 to 20 times with as much pressure as you can withstand; then switch to the other leg and do the same amount of repetitions. You will be amazed when you find out how many sore spots and lumps you have and did not even know it. Try to disintegrate those "bumps" you feel along the way. Or while you are watching TV, rub some arnica cream and begin rubbing those areas.

TIP #23:

When you are taking a shower, using soap, massage along the inner part of your forearm using your thumb. Start at the wrist and move toward the elbow. Do this 10 to 20 times with as much pressure as you can withstand; then switch to the other arm and do the same amount of repetitions. Or while watching TV, rub arnica cream and rub those areas.

TIP #24:

My stance: Cow milk is for cows, human milk is for babies. If you choose to drink cow milk, PLEASE PLEASE buy organic from pasture-raised animals. Buy any milk that does NOT have carrageenan, or better yet, make your own almond milk at home. Recipe follows. Carrageenan is making its way out of our markets (and it is carcinogenic.) See TIPS #77 and #204.

TIP #25:

Organic Almond Milk:
Soak one cup of organic almonds in water overnight. Make sure you add enough water for the almonds to absorb and expand. In the morning, drain the almonds but set the water aside. Blend the almonds with 4 cups of clean water. Strain through a nut milk bag. Blend the remaining pulp with 2 additional cups of water and strain through the nut milk bag. You can use the pulp for baking. The water you had overnight can be added to your plants; it gives them a special luster. See TIP #56.

TIP #26:

Thank Your God for the opportunity of a brand new day. Take ONE to TWO minutes and imagine how you want your day to be, intention is everything. Stage your day; make it as beautiful and as colorful as you wish. Remember, we all have trials and tribulations; the key lies on how we choose to see these trials and tribulations and how we choose to act upon them. AND (a big AND) how long we choose to hang on to them.
For example, picture the following scenario: "I wake up, jump out of bed, start rushing toward the bathroom; oops, I bang my little toe against the foot of the bed - I get angry, and I look at the mirror and do not like what I am seeing; then, as I shower I think of all the pendings I have at work, I get into my car (no time for breakfast), and rush through traffic; gosh, I hate traffic" and so on and so forth. What if you decide to picture your day as follows: I wake up, I stretch, I hug myself and say to myself: "What a great day, I am awake, I am alive, another opportunity to enjoy life. I have all the time in the world to get ready." I head toward the bathroom, oops I smash my little toe against the foot of the bed, I touch my toe and massage it, I see myself in the mirror and I smile back. I take a shower enjoying my body massage and the hot water.

I head down and grab a healthful breakfast bar. On my way to work I hit heavy traffic but I choose to enjoy music or listen to an audio-book while I drive to work. I decide today is made for me!!!! I give power to NO ONE! I CHOOSE to have a phenomenal day!" Can you feel the difference already? It is all about that inner talk you constantly have with yourself.

TIP #27:

Jell-O can come from the collagen in cow or pig bones and connective tissues. Nowadays the most common form of material used to make Jell-O is pigskin. In order for it to become powder, it needs to undergo several processes using strong acids or strong solvents to break the collagen down and then they pulverize it. I would rather avoid it.

TIP #28:

BONES are not supposed to crack!!!! Help them out by eating horsetail, nettle, and alfalfa in equal amounts. Use them in a powder and organic form and sprinkle on food or use in smoothies as often as possible. See TIP #100.

TIP #29:

Eat pomegranate, green tea, turmeric and broccoli. UK scientists from Bedford Hospital and Cambridge University Hospital show these super foods have proven to beat some cancers such as prostate. See TIPS #30 and #100.

TIP #30:

Turmeric is being considered the super-hero of the super-foods. It has anti-inflammatory properties, can inhibit tumor causing cells, supports the brain, can benefit diabetes, it is good for skin disorders, great antioxidant, helps tendonitis, joint pain, liver detoxification, any kind of arthritis, and so on. It can be used fresh, in a powder form or paste. I add it to my smoothie. See TIPS #12, #29, #100, #216, and #322.

TIP #31:

Beets: Add a 1" x 1" square of raw, peeled beet to your juice. It helps with circulation among other things. Cyclists use it in a powder form when riding long distances to enhance their breathing. Like anything, exercise caution. I used the powder once when doing yoga and it was too much for me; I started feeling dizzy. Raw beets, no problem. See TIPS #100 and #322.

TIP #32:

Have you heard of Ear Coning? It is an ancient technique used to pull the wax out of your ears. It has been used for over 2000 years by cultures such as Hindu, Tibetan, Chinese, Egyptian, Mayan, Aztec, and Incan. Nowadays, it is part of the curriculum of some European medical schools. It consists of a hollow cone, made out of cotton and covered with herbal oils and bee wax. You place it in your ear canal, while lying down on one side - and you light it. The smoke forms a suction and starts pulling out cerumen, fungus, spores, etc. Like anything, please be cautious and follow the instructions.

TIP #33:

Walking boosts brain chemistry into energy. It is best to walk very fast for about 5 or 10 minutes; then do it again several times throughout the day. It enhances your metabolism. Daily goal should be 10,000 steps or better. Help yourself: Park on the opposite side of the parking lot, use the stairs instead of the elevator, if you are waiting for someone walk around instead of sitting down, etc., etc., etc.. But, WALK!

TIP #34:

Coconut is great for the brain and it has multiple uses. I am talking about raw organic UNSWEETENED coconut in all its forms. Make desserts with raw organic shredded coconut, sprinkle it on food, put some in your smoothies or add some to yoghurt. Good quality coconut oil should have a white creamy consistency. See TIP #100.

TIP #35:

Eliminate REFINED sugar from your diet. Almost all processed products, canned or packaged, have refined sugar. It is labeled under different names: anything with the words sucrose, dextrose, cane sugar, brown sugar, cane crystals, corn sweetener, high fructose corn syrup, etc. is sugar. According to the movie "Fed-Up": sugar forces a reaction in your brain simulating cocaine. Once sugar enters your body, everything goes awry. It has also been linked to many types of cancers and behavioral issues in children. Next time you go to a children's party, check how they behave before and after you feed them sweets. See TIP #101 and TIP #5 for replacements.

TIP #36:

Sleeping is very important. You should sleep 7 to 9 hours every day. This is the time your body uses to regenerate itself. Less will carry you along for a while, but you need to be aware that you are in a constant state of depravation and it will catch up with you. We need to develop a relaxed environment: no iPads, no TV, no iPhones, no tablets, no clock lights, no lights from buttons from any device, at least 30 minutes before bed time. Try to go to bed 15 to 30 minutes before turning the lights off so your body can start slowing down; you might want to read a relaxed book or listen to something soothing. See TIP #55.

TIP #37:

There is plenty of research where it states that your second brain is your gut. As a matter of fact, research this title: "The Gut, Your Second Brain". Take care of it by ingesting fermented foods. Start simple: sauerkraut. No sugar, no additives. Just water, salt, and cabbage. At least 6 tbsp a day. There are many videos out there on how to make your own. Just make sure you add nothing other than salt and water. Or buy some already made. My favorite brand is Bubbies. Some fermented foods are kimchee, sauerkraut (just salt and water added; no other ingredient), kefir (coconut or seed based), miso, non-dairy yoghurt, kombucha.

TIP #38:

Whenever you feel stressed throughout the day, lock yourself in a quiet place (the bathroom works for me) for 3 to 5 minutes and breathe deeply, hug yourself, and tell yourself: "TODAY IS MADE FOR ME!!" or better yet "BE

STILL AND KNOW THAT I AM GOD-MADE". Repeat this constantly, sssslllllooooooowwwwwllllyyyyy, several times and keep on breathing. You will feel renewed and will be able to handle any situation in a more logical way.

TIP #39:

Check all labels in all the products you use on you and at home: nothing with parabens. They mimic hormones and have been found in breast cancer tumors in both, men and women. Replace one item at a time on a monthly basis until you have changed all products you use on your body and at home. See TIPS #208 (for product suggestions) and #287.

TIP #40:

Check the labels, nothing with sulfates since they are known to mimic hormones. Replace one item at a time on a monthly basis until you have changed all products you use on your body and at home. For product suggestion see TIPS #208 and #287.

TIP #41:

Ginger has many qualities. It is considered to be a fantastic energy booster. Add a 1" x 1" piece of ginger to your smoothie. See TIPS #100 and #322.

TIP #42:

Talking about exercise, I have never been an outdoorsy person nor one who enjoys exercise. When I am all gong ho, I enroll in these 1-hour programs of you name it: aqua aerobics, yoga, pilates, zumba, etc., and I do not last. I might stick with them for 1 or 2 years and kaput, finito! It is simply not my thing. See, when it comes to exercise, or anything in life for that matter, you need to be honest with yourself. I am not an exercise adept. BUT I HAVE DECIDED that I need to be active, my body deserves to be healthy, so **I found a wonderful program which lasts only 15 minutes a day (any one should have 15 minutes a day to themselves - if not, rearrange your schedule, you are too busy!) and it is called T-tapp. As the producer says: her specialty is "fitting fitness into your life rather than your life around your fitness program." It is a _mindful_ movement and low-impact exercise program customized to lose inches fast and build bone mass, which is what makes people excited. You do it for 21 days straight, and then graduate to the Total Workout and other more advanced workouts if you choose to. This has been my stick-to-it-veness exercise program. See TIPS #135, #139, and #140.**

TIP #43:

Dark spots on face and décolleté?
Use the juice of a lemon at night, let it dry and leave it on overnight. The following night, boil some rice until the rice is almost disintegrated. Keep the water refrigerated for about a week, at the most, and spread some of this water throughout the area to treat. Let it dry and leave it on overnight.
Alternate each night: one night use lemon juice, the following night use rice water. Make sure you use a sun block in the morning before you leave home. See TIP #237.

TIP #44:

Use a small brush to brush your fingernails and cuticle while you are bathing. When you come out of the shower, push your cuticle back with a wooden stick. The more you cut your cuticle, the more it will grow back. Cuticle is made to protect us. Put some vitamin E oil, jojoba oil, or coconut oil around the cuticle to keep it soft and smooth and rub some on your nails to make them shiny.

TIP #45:

Use a small brush to brush your toenails (different from the one you use for your fingernails) while you are bathing. When you come out of the shower, push your cuticle back with a wooden stick and add coconut oil, jojoba oil, or vitamin E on your toenails and feet.

TIP #46:

To prevent fungus in nails, gently file your nails on the top part to make them a bit porous, and then soak them in raw organic apple cider vinegar with the mother for about 10 minutes. Then dip a cotton ball with colloidal silver and soak your nail with it. It is very important to use a new cotton ball for each nail. If symptoms persist, consult your doctor.

TIP #47:

Coconut dessert:
Mix raw organic shredded unsweetened coconut, maple syrup, almond milk, and walnuts. Enjoy! Fast, quick and a healthful concoction.

TIP #48:

Use exfoliating gloves to cleanse your body and to increase circulation when you are taking a shower.

Always try to cleanse yourself in a circular motion and toward the heart. Remember to change the gloves every 3 to 6 months.

TIP #49:

There have been many recent investigations about gluten. Gluten has always been in our food supply. The difference is that nowadays the gluten content on the products we consume is so condensed that it makes it unable to digest it. Some individuals may be more sensitive than others, but my position is: eat as less gluten as possible. There are many products which are gluten-free but make sure they don't have added sugar in them. There is an incredible enzyme on the market that helps you process gluten too. See TIP #286.

TIP #50:

There is a link between hemorrhoids and sitting in the water room for a while. So, if you are one of those who reads in that special room, STOP! If you do have hemorrhoids, take warm water baths with aloe vera. Sit for 15 to 20 minutes. If symptoms persist, consult a physician.

TIP #51:

Cravings are very smart mechanisms which your body utilizes to let you know there is an imbalance in your body. An occasional craving, now and then, is okay. Pay attention to what you crave: sugar, salt, etc. and if your cravings are constant. This means you are lacking something in your diet or you cannot digest what you are eating. Enzymes will help you balance this.

TIP #52:

If you enjoy granola make your own:
1/2 cup of steel-cut oatmeal
1/4 cup each: almonds, chopped apples, chopped pears
1/4 cup unsweetened shredded coconut
Cashew or almond milk
Maple syrup or honey to taste

Directions:
Boil 2 cups of water.
Add oatmeal and cook for about 7 to 10 minutes.
Drain oatmeal.
Add fruit, almonds, coconut, and milk to oatmeal.
Sweeten to taste.

Substitute apples and pears for:
Strawberries, raspberries, blueberries, and/or blackberries.
Peaches

TIP #53:

Bad breath? A great mouth refresher after a meal or
between meals is "Mint Assure". It is a combination of
parsley and mint.   But if it is a continuous thing, you need to
see what is wrong with your digestion and/or your teeth and
gums.

TIP #54:

MORNING ROUTINE

**I start the day with a glass or two of water as soon as I
wake up.**
**I take enzymes to support my heart, eyes, and energy
levels.**

I pet my gorgeous cats, about 5 minutes each one.
I take bee pollen or royal jelly.
I exercise 20 to 50 minutes.
Prepare my smoothie - TIP #100 - (sometimes my green juice - TIP #12) and my lunch.
Take digestive enzymes, probiotics, and biotin with either: 1) a small apple and 6 cashews; 2) alfalfa with sauerkraut; 3) 1/2 protein bar - TIP #213.
Get ready for the day.
Drink my smoothie.

TIP #55:

It is important to go to bed at the same time every day, whatever that may be for you depending on your work schedule. You need to go to bed and wake up at the same time every day. This will regulate melatonin production and train your brain to be alert when you need it to be. See TIP #36.

TIP #56:

If you eat almonds, they should be raw, preferably; and always, always soak them overnight and wash them before you eat them. The skin of almonds is an enzyme inhibitor. See TIPS #25 and #100.

TIP #57:

Cut 1"x1" pieces of eggplant and soak in water overnight. Strain and drink water throughout the day as a preventative measure for high cholesterol.

TIP #58:

Grape Seed Extract is an incredible antioxidant which can help with collagen production and bone strength, brain support, and enhances wound healing. See TIP #100.

TIP #59:

Maca is a wonderful superfood. It helps with energy, stamina, memory, and it helps your adrenals. Just add 1/2 teaspoon or so to your morning smoothie. Make sure your source is a qualified one. If you are breast-feeding or pregnant or if you have any hormone-sensitive condition, avoid its use. See TIP #100.

TIP #60:

Recipe for Mouthwash:

2 cups of food-grade oxygen peroxide
1 1/2 teaspoons of aluminum-free baking soda
1/3 cup of a fluoride-free mouthwash (I use Neem Mouthwash)
2 tablespoons of Colloidal silver
It is very important to use food-grade oxygen peroxide.

TIP #61:

Aloe Vera is one of the most incredibly skin soothing divine remedies: Use the real plant. Cut a strip through the middle and use the juice of the cactus directly on the skin and let it dry. It is fantastic for rashes, acne, skin care, baby rash, radiation-treated skin (after it dries, you rub a good quality moisturizing cream - that is what I did with my belated husband and it worked), sunburns, frost bites, mosquito repellent or baby diaper rash. If you are going to purchase it, I would make sure it is, at least, 98% organic aloe vera. I love "Skin Gel" from Aloe Life.

TIP #62:

Microwaves heat food by causing water molecules to turn into steam which, in turn, heats your food. This is why food is heated so fast, but what people fail to realize is that it causes a chemical change in your food. I understand that due to everyday living it is impossible not to use it. Do your best to use the microwave oven as little as possible because it kills ALL the nutritional value in your food. I use it as storage at home.

TIP #63:

According to Harvard Health "………**There is no single substance called plastic.** That term covers many materials made from an array of organic and inorganic compounds. Substances are often added to plastic to help shape or stabilize it. Two of these plasticizers are
- bisphenol-A (BPA), added to make clear, hard plastic
- phthalates, added to make plastic soft and flexible

BPA and phthalates are believed to be 'endocrine disruptors.' These are substances that mimic human hormones, and not for the good.
When food is wrapped in plastic or placed in a plastic container and microwaved, BPA and phthalates may leak into the food."
So, bottom line, PLEASE make sure your plastic containers have a microwave-safe label or just use glass containers. See TIP #66.

TIP #64:

On the same line of TIP #63, I do not buy anything with phthalates. Remember, phthalates mimic hormones, so I am very careful when buying cosmetics, lotions, etc. Read the labels. There are several options for cosmetics. If you want to learn more, check the cosmetic database from the Environmental Work Group. See TIP #287.

TIP #65:

Replace your old pots and pans if they have a non-stick surface, commonly known as teflon. Get stainless steel pots and pans instead. According to the Environmental Working Group, toxic fumes released from your teflon-coated pots and pans may cause flu-like symptoms or may even kill birds. Imagine the havoc this could play in our bodies due to the accumulation of years cooking with them. See TIPS #63, #66, and #268.

TIP #66:

Make a commitment with yourself and purchase one pot/pan on odd months until they are all replaced and buy one glass container on even months to substitute all your plastic containers. Plastic containers are okay as long as you DO NOT use them to heat things. See TIPS #63, #65 and #268.

TIP #67:

Facial Scrub
Courtesy from Organic Gardening:

1 Cup Rolled Oats

1/3 Cup Cornmeal
1/3 Cup Dried Peppermint (or herb of choice)

Grind all ingredients to a fine powder.
Store into a tightly sealed container for up to 3 months.
Place a small amount on your hand and add enough water
to form a paste.
Massage gently over your face and rinse thoroughly. It is a
bit messy so I do it in the shower.

TIP #68:

**Tapping is also known as EFT (Emotional Freedom
Technique). It is a simple and revolutionary technique
for emotional self-improvement. It is a mixture of
different disciplines: acupressure, meditation, and
modern psychology. It is fast and you can sometimes
feel immediate results. You can improve your health,
relationships, well-being, and much more. If you are
interested check the Tapping Solution. I use it all the
time.**

TIP #69:

Beans are a great source of fiber and protein. Many
individuals dislike them because they cause flatulence. To
avoid that, you need to soak them for about 48 hours
changing the water 2 to 3 times a day. That foamy water is
what causes flatulence. Rinse them thoroughly and cook
them slowly. Doctor them up with fried onion, garlic, and sea
or Himalayan salt. Add chopped herbs such as parsley,
cilantro, epazote. And doll them up with some cashewgurt!

TIP #70:

Radishes are a great food when you have cravings or when you are very hungry. Just try it: eat one or two radishes before your main meal and they will calm your appetite.

TIP #71:

Bee Pollen is one of the most complete foods out there. It has the perfect amount of protein, carbohydrates, fat, and minerals. Just make sure it comes from bees instead of plants. It boosts your energy too. Take one teaspoon in the morning with breakfast. Make sure you are not allergic to it. See TIP #11.

TIP #72:

Try to get a hair color which is ammonia-free. Ammonia could be deadly if ingested. According to the U. S. National Library of Medicine some known symptoms are: cough, chest pain, chest tightness, difficulty breathing, wheezing, rapid breathing, fever, rapid/weak pulse, dizziness, lack of coordination, lip swelling, mouth pain, burning of eyes among others. In this day and age it is very difficult to live a chemical-free life, but the less chemicals we use, the better off we will be.

TIP #73:

Colloidal Silver is one of the most diverse products available to us, and one of my favorite. I have drank it when I have a sore throat, and I have used it as a general house cleaner as well. And anything in between: to clean wounds, colds, abrasions, rashes, de-parasitic, acne-prone skin, minor eye

infections, etc. There are different concentrations and
purities so it requires due diligence.

TIP #74:

For colds or sore throats (without fever) I use different things:
- One teaspoon each of organic Ceylon cinnamon and raw
  honey. If you have a sensitive stomach, this is not for
  you; cinnamon can irritate it. Make a paste and rub it in
  the back of the throat.
-   Mixture of the following ingredients: 1 cup of food-grade
  hydrogen peroxide, 4 tablespoons of colloidal silver, 1
  tablespoon of aluminum-free baking soda. Mix it very well
  and gargle with it.
- Boil 3 garlic cloves, one stick of Ceylon cinnamon, and
  water. Pour the hot water in a cup and add lemon and
  honey. Drink as hot as possible.
- Gargle with simple Isodine. See TIPS #148, #157, #176,
  and #211.

Tip #75:

Here is a recipe for shea butter, and extremely easy to
make! A small amount goes a long way. I use it on my
hands and feet; it is truly fantastic! You will need a dedicated
pot for it, a wooden spoon, and a glass jar along with the
following ingredients:
1/4 cup Beeswax (raw, organic preferably)
3/4 cup Coconut Oil (raw, organic preferably)
3/4 cup Coconut Butter (raw, organic preferably)
1/3 cup Shea Butter (organic)
1 teaspoon each of Vitamin E, Jojoba Oil, and Almond Oil
2 teaspoons Essential Oil of your choice (I usually use
Lavender)

In a dedicated pot on low heat, melt the beeswax very slowly and stir continuously. Once it is completely melted, add the coconut oil, coconut butter, and shea butter. Stir non-stop until they melt. Take away from heat and add the other ingredients right away. Pour in jar(s) immediately before it solidifies. See TIP #**299**.

TIP #76:

Produce labeling can be very confusing. The numbers appearing on fruits and vegetables actually mean something. The following information might help you decipher them:
PLU stands for 'Price Look Up.'
If it starts with a '3' or '4' = It means it has been conventionally grown. This encompasses the use of chemicals and pesticides so goods can grow faster, bigger, and last longer.
If it starts with an 8 = It means those goods are genetically engineered, which translates to goods which have been engineered by a machine or a human. Avoid them at all costs.
If it starts with a '9' = it means it is organic. Organic means that the soil that touched the good has not been chemically treated by pesticides, herbicides, fertilizers or antibiotics. But beware: some of the skins are treated with wax so they do not bruise during transportation so rinse them well. See TIPS #20, #21, #225, #**241,** and #306.

TIP #77:

Carrageenan is in many products including milk, yoghurt, and many others. There is a polemic going on about this ingredient. Some have linked it to certain types of cancer and it is slowly making its way out of the market. I avoid anything with it. See TIP #24.

TIP #78:

Ghee is clarified butter. It has been separated from the milk through low heat. What is left is just the fat, no milk residue. It is a good source of Omega 3's. It is a basic food in Ayurvedic foods but use it sparingly since it is fat, a good source, but fat nonetheless. See TIP #81.

TIP #79:

Meditation is a handy tool to use when we are experiencing stressful events or stressful moments in our lives. And by stressful I mean positive as well as negative experiences in life. The majority of individuals believe that you focus your mind in one object while your body relaxes and your mind unwinds, and that could probably be the most popular type, but there are many other types. Some resonate with a specific mantra tailored to their vibrations in a sitting position. Others just repeat a mantra over and over again while walking in a labyrinth or just walking, etc. Others follow guided meditations. **Regardless of which avenue you choose, it is good to meditate even if it is only for minutes a day.**

TIP #80:

The perfect solution for soft, smooth skin is coconut oil. I purchase an organic raw coconut oil (I use Artisana) and use it all over my skin about twice a month after showering depending on how dry my skin feels and the time of year. Add a couple tablespoons to your bath; use it as facial cream too. What a better way to be as chemical-free as possible and quite inexpensive too.

TIP #81:

Butter vs Margarine
Margarine is an artificial concoction and should not be eaten.
Our body is not configured to digest it. If you have to eat it,
choose organic butter from pasture-raised cows, free of
antibiotics. See TIP #78.

TIP #82:

I use toothpastes which have neem or tea tree oil as their
main ingredient. There are many options out there. There is
aluminum-free baking soda toothpaste too.   See TIPS #8,
#60, and #202.

TIP #83:

Superfoods are the most powerful, nutritious, mineral-rich
plant foods on Earth. They are essential for our well-being.
Superfoods immediately nourish the brain, bones, muscles,
skin, hair, nails, heart, lungs, liver, kidneys, reproductive
system, pancreas, and most importantly the immune system.
In the long-term, superfoods help correct imbalances
because they provide maximum nutrition. Consuming
superfoods makes it much easier to achieve ideal weight
and follow healthy food habits. For those who believe that
health is a priority, smoothies should be a significant part of
your day. See TIP #100.

TIP #84:

 Our present lifestyle is surrounded and bombarded with
chemicals. In this day and age we will never be able to lead
a chemical-free life; therefore, we need to be conscious of
what surrounds us and try to eliminate as many chemicals

as possible in order to live a healthier and longer life. One widely trend is the use of plug-ins. They have Volatile Organic Compounds (VOC's) which are highly toxic. Use diffusers with essential oils instead.

TIP #85:

Celery Root is a wonderful root vegetable. It has magnesium, calcium, iron, and potassium. It also has vitamin C as well as several of the B vitamins. Cook it as you cook potatoes and add it to eggs, for example.

TIP #86:

Massage between the nose and the upper lip with your index finger. It regulates the appetite and reduces stress.

TIP #87:

Chia seeds are among one of the healthiest foods available to us. They need to be soaked overnight in order for our body to utilize all their nutritional value. Soak one cup of chia seeds to 5 cups of water. If you want to use chia seeds for puddings use 4 cups of water instead. See TIPS #100 and #206.

TIP #88:

Quinoa is a nutritious grain known for its great protein content, but even more for the type of protein which has all 9 essential amino acids plus iron. It comes in different colors: red, black, and white. Boil it or cook it as you would rice and eat it cold or hot. Add it to salads, soups, etc.

TIP #89:

Colon Hydrotherapy, also known as colonics, is a clean and comfortable treatment which will relieve constipation and maintain healthy bowel regimen. A gentle flow of warm water is introduced into the colon which stimulates the natural peristaltic motion of the colon and the individual will naturally evacuate during the process. This is a very gentle experience. I do this once every 2 to 3 years, but ALWAYS CONSULT A PHYSICIAN for any health concerns you may have.

TIP #90:

Physical exercise is known to reduce the risk of cardiovascular disease, and now researchers have observed that regular exercise can reduce the blood pressure in the eyes as well as improve blood flow to the retina. Additionally, individuals who spend more time outdoors have a reduced risk of macular degeneration. (Journal of Glaucoma, June 2016). This is another reason to exercise!!!!

TIP #91:

Coconut Pudding:
1 cup chia seeds (soaked overnight in 2 to 3 cups of water)
2 cups raw shredded coconut
3 tsps vanilla extract
1 cup pecans (finely chopped)
Maple syrup to taste

Drain chia seeds if there is any water left.
Blend all ingredients (except pecans) in food processor
Fold pecans and refrigerate overnight
Compliments of Ritamarie Loscalzo

TIP #92:

Cordyceps and Reishi Mushrooms are great for the endocrine system. They help in aiding adrenal fatigue and they support the thyroid. You can find them in the form of organic powders. See TIPS #100, #187, #193, #249, #257, #281, #342, #345, and #352.

TIP #93:

Pomegranate powder may soothe burning from acid reflux; it has an alkaline effect when ingested in the form of tea. It is a great antioxidant too. See TIPS #29 and #100.

TIP # 94:

Eat blueberries often. They boost brain power, heart, skin, sight, and overall support to your immune system - See TIP #100.

TIP #95:

If you are a carnivore, make your own deli meats. Cook a turkey or a chicken (preferably organic and grass-fed or pasture-raised) or whatever you fancy and then slice it; let it cool down. Separate it in small amounts and wrap them in the following order: Place the meat in saran wrap, then plastic wrap, and lastly aluminum foil, and freeze them; they will last for months. Make sure that when you thaw one package you eat it. You may refrigerate it for up to 2 days but you should not freeze it again. Processed meats have high sodium content, preservatives, coloring, etc.

TIP #96:

Table salt (white refined salt) is added to many foods to enhance their flavor and it is a highly processed food. Salt is linked to hypertension. Avoid prepared foods and packaged foods, and definitely canned foods - they are all usually very high in sodium even if the label says 'low in sodium.' When you go out to restaurants always order your dish with "no added salt". Use sea salt or Himalayan salt but use it sparingly; salt is salt but at least you are not ingesting chemicals. See TIP #97.

TIP #97:

Here is a list of what herbs and spices to use with what foods in order to enhance their flavor (instead of salt):
Beef - Marjoram, orange rind, lemon rind, sage, thyme.
Broccoli/Cauliflower - Dill, cumin, curry powder, lemon juice, oregano, parsley.
Carrots, onions - Dill, marjoram, rosemary, sage.
Chicken - Rosemary, sage, parsley and lemon, tarragon, thyme.
Fish - Curry powder, dill seed, dill weed, lemon, mustard, rosemary, sage, tarragon, thyme.
Green beans - Dill, lemon juice, onion, oregano, parsley, pepper.
Quinoa - Black garlic, epazote
Potato - Chives, curry powder, dill, pepper, rosemary.
Tomatoes - Basil, bay leaf, cilantro, dill, onion, oregano, parsley.
Zucchini - Oregano, parsley.
Be creative. Try new herbs. Your mind is the limit! See TIP #96.

TIP #98:

Individuals who are allergic to some foods have compromised their immune system to a point where the body starts attacking itself when they continue eating the foods they are allergic to. They might have developed a short list of foods to choose from but, eventually, that list will start getting shorter and shorter. Those individuals will reach a point when they will even react to good food, a point of no return unless they change their eating habits. See TIPS #141, #266, and #314.

TIP #99:

Regardless of what faith or spiritual practice you come from, the more individuals pray, the better off we are. Form prayer circles, form groups where each one of the members pray at the same time from the comfort of their own home, pray together as a family, etc. The power of words and thoughts have an impact at a vibrational level.

TIP #100:

My recipe for a green smoothie:
See TIPS #14, #28, #29, #30, #31, #34, #41, #56, #58, #59, #83, #87, #92, #93, #94, #129, #143, #257, #272, #322, #326, #336, #362, and #375.
The ratio should be 2/3 greens and 1/3 fruits.
1 leaf of romaine lettuce
1 leaf of mustard greens
1 leaf of red and green Swiss chard
1 leaf of collard greens
2 handful of power greens
1 handful of spinach
Some others I use are: Dandelion leaves, arugula, kale, etc.

1/8 to 1/4 tsp each of the following powders: cordyceps, reishi, pomegranate, horsetail, maca, nettle, alfalfa, açai, chlorella, moringa leaf, ashwagandha, astragalus, chaga, spirulina, grape seed extract (powder), marine collagen peptides

1 cube each (1" x 1" appx) of fresh ginger, fresh turmeric, fresh carrot, fresh coconut, and fresh beet.

4 to 6 goji berries

raw unsweetened coconut

1/2 tsp of flaxseed

1/2 tsp of soaked chia (overnight)

1/2 tsp hemp seeds

1 scoop of a RAW well-balanced protein powder

1 Brazilian nut (which is all the omega 6 you need in one day)

(I interchange the nuts with 2 or 3 of either raw organic pecans, cashews, almonds or walnuts).

The combination of fruits I use are as follows: Strawberries, cranberries, blueberries, blackberries, raspberries, and cherries (all organic), and one date.

1/2 organic fuji apple and 1/2 organic pear

1 organic thin pineapple slice and 2 kiwis

4 kiwis

The juice of 1 grapefruit and 1 pear

1 plum and 1 peach

You can do as many combinations as you wish, just try to choose low-glycemic fruits more often than not.

BY THE WAY, I did not start this way. I started mixing some romaine, butter, or other type of lettuce with some spinach and flaxseeds, and lots and lots of water with fruit. I increased my greens and powders as I got used to the flavor.

TIP #101:

Stop ingesting anything that is fat-free or light. The producers of these items load them with sugar so they can taste better but you will end up with unwanted pounds plus you are ingesting chemicals. Since the invention and introduction of fat-free and low-fat items in the US market and around the world, people have gained more weight than ever. Check out the documentary "Fed-Up." See TIPS #5 and #35.

TIP #102:

Colas are a NO NO, especially dark sodas. They have zero nutritional value and they are full of dyes and loaded with sugar among other things; and that includes those horrendous energy drinks. Read the ingredients, they have some you cannot even pronounce. Try to replace one soda a day for flavored fresh water: add slices of cucumber and parsley; orange slices, grapefruit slices, etc. or drink green tea. It is a fantastic way to shed pounds too.

TIP #103:

We need to have a balance between Omega 3's and Omega 6's. We usually eat way too many omega 6's. Good sources fo Omega 3's are cold water fish such as tuna, salmon, and halibut. A good combo of Omega 3's and 6's are sunflower seeds and flaxseeds; add these seeds to your salads or to your smoothies.

TIP #104:

Let's make us aware here: Do cars run without gasoline?????? THEY DO NOT and it works the same for you body: YOUR BODY NEEDS BREAKFAST. Plan on it. Have some nuts and a sliced apple, eggs (organic and pasture-raised), smoothies, etc.

TIP #105:

Test your pH. Our bodies do best when we have a pH between 6.5 and 7 (pH ranges from 1 to 14). Purchase simple test strips at your local market. You can use these strips to measure the pH in your saliva and in your urine. The best way to test it is first thing upon awakening before you even drink water and the first urination of the day. Remember, our aim is between 6.5 and 7. This is the range where all minerals get absorbed. See TIP#205.

TIP #106:

The nutritional value of your food disappears as you cook it. Anything cooked over 110 F (43 C) has lost some nutritional value. The ideal thing is to get, at least, 50% of your food intake from raw food but I understand this could be hard for some of us so you need to help your body break down and assimilate the food you are eating, even if it is good food. You accomplish this by taking digestive enzymes with every single meal and snack, at first bite. There are specific good-quality enzymes which will help digest carbs, fats, dairy, gluten, protein, etc. See TIPS #49, #54, #142, #155, #160, 207, #219, #222, #276, #310, #319, #320, and #346.

TIP #107:

A difference exists between folate and folic acid. Folate is an essential nutrient found in leafy greens and folic acid is a synthetic compound which oxidizes in your body and it is found in many processed foods. It has been linked to deterioration of cognitive function in adults.

TIP #108:

Don't drink or eat anything at least two hours before going to bed. This will help your stomach settle and avoid acidity.

TIP #109:

Cabbage is an excellent food; besides being very filling, it is low caloric so you can have unlimited amounts. It is an excellent source of beta carotene which is good for your eye sight, it improves brain function, and reduces the build up in your arteries supporting your heart and lowering your blood pressure. It is a great source of probiotics if fermented properly.

TIP #110:

Regarding your deodorant, try to use one that has no aluminum. Aluminum has been linked to breast cancer in, both, men and women. There are rocks and sprays that you can use instead.

TIP #111:

Just because it says natural on the front label of a product DOES NOT mean it is good for you. Many harmful things for the human body are natural. ALWAYS read the ingredients on the label and avoid anything that says 'natural flavors' unless the manufacturer specifies the source and it is something healthful. See TIPS #287 and #308.

TIP #112:

Triclosan is an ingredient added to many products to reduce bacterial contamination: soaps, body washes, etc. There are some on-going studies which suggest the possibility of making bacteria resistant with continuous use of triclosan. I believe soap and water will do the trick as long as you wash your hands and rub your nails thoroughly for 15 to 20 seconds.

TIP #113:

According to a Harvard study, your posture can affect your muscle production. Your ear, shoulder, hip, knee, and ankle should be in a straight line when you see yourself from the side. When sitting down you should keep even weight on your feet. To learn exercises to improve your posture check Harvard Health and search under posture and back health.

TIP #114:

Your skin is the largest organ in your body. Treat it accordingly. Use products that do not have any coloring: Blue #5, Yellow #3, Red #7; phthalates, parabens, fragrance, etc. Did you know that companies do not have to disclose what ingredients they use to add fragrance to items? See TIP #287.

TIP #115:

Clothes touch your skin. The laundry soap you use to wash them should be as natural as possible: Try to get a no-fragrance, no parabens, no sulfates soap. See TIP #287.

TIP #116:

The best diet:
As one of my teachers used to say: The best diet is one "i",
one "i": ONE ITEM, ONE INGREDIENT. In other words,
fresh whole fruits and vegetables, organic if possible; grains,
pasture-raised meats, organic chicken, wild-caught fish.
Nothing fried or breaded! See TIPS #20 and #21.

TIP #117:

Add glycerin oil to your body lotions to add even more
moisture.

TIP #118:

The American Optometric Association recommends taking
frequent breaks when using smart phones, tablets or
computers if used over long periods of time; if not, you might
experience headaches, blurred vision, dry eyes, and neck or
shoulder pain. This syndrome is called computer vision or
digital eye strain.

TIP #119:

There are certain things that might help if you experience
migraines:
Caffeine, feet in cold water, and Niacin (no-flush) help blood
flow to the brain.

TIP #120:

Bee stings can be very painful. If the victim is allergic please
take him/her to the Emergency. Otherwise, extract the liquid

by pulling the skin and pressing down. Follow by washing the area with clean cold water. Make a poultice with bread, milk, and honey and put over sting pressing it down with a fork. This will help with the pain and inflammation.

TIP #121:

Problems with mosquitoes during the summer? Try planting basil, a natural mosquito deterrent; they do not like the aroma. Or use citronella candles. See TIPS #227, #255, #360, and #367.

TIP #122:

Do you suffer from constipation?
A quick remedy:
A couple of tablespoons of olive oil, and make a habit of drinking cabbage juice.

TIP #123:

Olive oil (cold pressed preferably) is a very good source to use COLD; when heated it changes its nutritional value. Use it as a salad dressing, scattered on toast instead of butter, etc. See TIP #124.

TIP #124:

Basic salad dressing:
1/4 lemon
1/4 cup of olive oil (cold pressed preferably)
Pinch of sea salt or Himalayan salt
Mix well and coat lightly.

To this, you can add any herb to flavor it: dill, rosemary, basil, mint, etc.

TIP #125:

Oils which are polyunsaturated have omega 6's and omega 3's making them good choices for cooking such as coconut oil. A good monounsaturated oil to cook with is avocado oil. Keep them in a cool, dry, and dark place.

TIP #126:

Among the worst oils to cook with are seed-based oils and canola oil (used in Canadian refineries). Canola oil needs to be 100% organic if you are to ingest it.

TIP #127:

Job's tears (also known as Chinese pearl barley, Coix, or Adlay millet) is a gluten-free grain high in protein. It has a chewy, nutty texture. It could be used instead of hominy or garbanzo and it is cooked just like rice although Job's tears will not absorb the water, they need to be drained. They could be used in soups, salads, main dishes; imagination is unlimited. Individuals taking diabetic medications should be careful as it lowers blood sugar.

TIP #128:

Chlorophyll is another super food. It has many benefits: It might help control hunger and cravings, alleviate constipation, promote cleansing, and it might be effective against candida. Add it to your smoothie.

TIP #129:

Moringa leaf is a natural energy booster, high in vitamin C, B2, B6, and magnesium. According to "Pure Healing Foods" it is known "to lower blood pressure and the leafs are a natural vitamin providing 7 x the vitamin C of oranges, 4 x the calcium of milk, 4 x the vitamin A of carrots, 3 x the potassium of bananas, and 2 x the protein of yoghurt." See TIP #100

TIP #130:

Do you suffer from constipation?
Try this breakfast to aid your elimination:
Steel-cut oatmeal
2 teaspoons of flaxseed
4 pitted prunes
Apple or pear
Water
And chew, chew, chew.

TIP #131:

Hand salve:
8 oz (224 ml) lavender infused or almond oil
1 oz (28 grams) beeswax (grated)
4 capsules of vitamin 'E'
10 drops lavender essential oil (or your choice)
10 drops rosemary

In a pot, pour lavender infused oil and heat on low.
Add beeswax and stir until it fully melts.
Remove pot from heat and add the rest of the ingredients.
Pour in a glass container and let it cool.
Store in a cool place for up to one year. See TIP #299.

TIP #132:

Always be very mindful of washing your hands to avoid colds, especially during flu season (in the US - October thru March). Wash them for 15 to 20 seconds, grab a paper towel and close the handle with the paper towel. Throw it away and grab another one to dry your hands, and open the door with that towel, then throw it away. These steps will save you from several colds. See TIPS #144, #148, #211, and #215.

TIP #133:

Garlic is a natural antibiotic and a substitute for aspirin. It is an excellent supporter of your respiratory, circulatory, and digestive systems. Its natural ingredient, sulphur, can be found in nails, hair, and skin. One way to ingest it is by mincing a garlic clove and swallowing it with a bit of liquid. If you choose to take pills instead of the garlic itself the pills should smell; if they don't, they will not help you; the key ingredient is sulphur.

TIP #134:

Phosphatidylserine is involved in many biological processes. Brain cells are rich in phosphatidylserine. There are very few studies that show if this substance can help with memory loss, but there are some clinical trials where they say that people who have had it experience less stress, and many believe that if you are free from stress you have a healthier brain.

TIP #135:

Pilates saved me from serious structural issues. When I was in my thirties I had many bone-related incidents: hip displacement, issues with ankles, back problems, and so on and so forth; they were constant and very painful. I ended up going to a TRUE - and I cannot emphasize this enough - a TRUE Pilates therapist. I found a place where professional personnel dedicated their lives to heal injured ballerinas and dancers. And I stress again: TRUE Pilates. They changed my life: within days they healed a hip displacement I had been dealing with for months and, after some one-to-one classes to strengthen my body, I transitioned to group classes which I took for about 1 year. No jumping, no exercises to pump the heart, etc. These fantastic therapists gave me a promising future. This was my first step toward structural health. See TIPS #42, #139, and #140.

TIP #136:

Salad bags help your leafy greens stay fresh longer, they double their life time! There are many different types to choose from. I use one which is made out of terrycloth material. The trick is you need to wash your leafy greens as soon as you get home from the market, let them drain and put them in the salad bag which is already moist; do not let the leafy greens dry. Make sure the salad bag remains moist so the veggies don't wilt and rot. I love mine! See TIP #322.

TIP #137:

Woke up with bags under your eyes? Are you going to a party and would like to look refreshed? COLD cucumber slices on your eyes for about 10 to 15 minutes. Or peel a white potato and grate it, then take two pieces of cotton and place the potato inside the cotton and place it on your eyes for 10 to 15 minutes.

TIP #138:

Magnesium: One of the most important minerals for your body. Have it tested! According to Natural Society "Serum or blood level measurements are usually inadequate because magnesium operates on a cellular level and accumulates in organ and nerve tissue. So even good results with blood testing are very often deceptive, leaving one with a magnesium deficiency. One effective test developed for use by health professionals is the "Exa Test." It is worth every penny! Some symptoms of magnesium deficiency are: Muscle cramps, anxiety, dizziness, fatigue, poor memory, poor heart health.

TIP #139:

Egoscue: Pete Egoscue a master of exercise. This is when I learnt that lots of "minor aches and pains" are because your bones are misaligned, they are structural dysfunctions. And with time, as we grow older, these minor discrepancies can lead us to serious structural issues and an inability to walk with ease. Egoscue helped me get rid of those annoying aches and pains which people believe to be normal as we grow in years. This was my second step toward structural health and toward a complete pain-free life style. See TIPS #42, #135, and #140.

TIP #140:

A way to keep your body aligned is through fascia release or massage. Fascia is the underlying mesh which surrounds your bones, nerves, blood vessels, and muscles. With repetitive daily movements we twist and turn this connective tissue and it changes our structure. Having a fascia massage every month or every quarter will keep you in top shape. See TIPS #42, #135, and #139.

TIP #141:

Do you suffer from allergies? Try avoiding these foods before trying anything else. These are the top 5 allergens:
Corn or corn related products
Peanuts
Soy
Wheat
Dairy
Stop all of them at the same time and after one month, try to introduce one item at a time for an entire week and watch your body, tune in to what you feel: Is your energy level the same, do you feel jittery, are you sleepy after you eat, slight headaches, any aches or pains, do you feel bloated, do you have an emotional upheaval several hours after eating, do your sinus act up, are your fingers swollen, do your joints hurt? If so, you are allergic to that one specific food. See TIPS #98, #266, and #314.

TIP #142:

Probiotics are live bacteria and yeast which are very beneficial to your gut. They should be taken daily and together with digestive enzymes is the best thing you can do for your digestion. There is a variety of foods available with probiotics: Yoghurt, kefir, fermented foods (naturally done - only water and salt added), Rejuvelac, or AT LEAST, a 7-billion probiotic. For those who are over 50, I love the raw 85-billion probiotic from Garden of Life. See TIPS #146 and #155.

TIP #143:

Astragalus is a root which has been used in China for centuries. It helps boost your immune system, helps with aging (it boosts the telomerase enzyme), and improves energy. It might increase the risk of bleeding so avoid it if you have any bleeding disorder. See TIP #100.

TIP #144:

For Flu season (October-March in the U.S.) start taking Echinacea and Propolis. Take 2 capsules 3 times a day for the first week; 2 capsules twice a day for the second week; 2 capsules once a day for the rest of the season through the end of March. See TIPS #132, #148, #211, and #215.

TIP #145:

Start your meals by blessing your food. It will relax you and it will provide the right environment to unwind your digestive system and allow the food to be properly digested, absorbed, transported, and eliminated, all parts of digestion.

TIP #146:

Rejuvelac is a cultured probiotic-rich drink made by fermenting freshly sprouted grains in water. It is a slight-tart, lemony-tasting liquid as digestive aid to increase enzyme content in the diet. Start slowly by drinking 2 to 4 teaspoons at a time. Be cautious: You need to use clean soapy water to clean all jars, spoons, lids, etc. It can go bad easily! See TIP #142.

TIP #147:

Bitter melon, when consumed in raw or juice form can lower glucose levels but does not significantly reduce A1C.

TIP #148:

Use a nasal spray as a regular routine to cleanse your nasal passages. There is a wide variety to choose from and they do not require prescription. Pump two sprays in each nostril, do not inhale; let it come out and gently blow your nose. Use it every day once a day to keep your nose nice, clean, and healthy. If you have a cold or suffer from allergies use it 3 to 6 times a day or even more if need be. There are some nasal sprays which contain manganese and I have found them very helpful. The one I use is Sterimar. See TIPS #74, #132, #144, #157, #176, and #211.

TIP #149:

Do you suffer from headaches?
Home remedy:
Avoid processed food, sugar, and grains.
Smell Peppermint or Winter Green Essential Oil.
Use enzymes to lower frequency and intensity. See TIP #242.

TIP #150:

Biotin is also known as Vitamin B7, B8, or Vitamin H. It helps metabolize fats, carbs, and amino-acids. It also transforms glucose into energy and keeps our tissue cells healthy such as the skin, hair, and nails. Black currant seed oil and zinc are great too. I take one

capsule of Biotin every day every other month. I do not take combination products; just straight biotin.

TIP #151:

Do you suffer from bunions? Dr. Scholl has a gadget you can wear at night; it is excellent and inexpensive. It pulls your big toe and aligns it. Try to do this before the bone starts protruding. I wear them when the bone starts bothering me.

TIP #152:

There is a tiny book out there from Emmet Fox: 40-day Prosperity Plan. Great tiny easy-read book. Highly recommend it!

TIP #153:

Coffee is not bad for everyone. Pay attention to your body: If you feel sleep deprived or anxious maybe coffee is not good for you and you need to eliminate it from your diet. For those of you who do not have any side effects you need to know that coffee undergoes several chemical steps; the coffee that our grandparents drank is not the same as the one we drink. If you cannot give up caffeine, then get a water-processed based coffee; this will be your best choice.

TIP #154:

When I was a teenager a man who worked for Lancôme told me to use glycerin on my eyelashes for them to grow; he said I would remember him for the rest of my life. I have not been very consistent..........but I do remember him. See TIP #159.

TIP #155:

Do you suffer from peptic or intestinal ulcers or gastritis? According to an article in "Applied and Environmental Microbiology" they identified a strain of probiotic bacteria called Bifidobacterium bifidum which helps to decrease ulcers and stomach conditions such as gastritis. All probiotics are not created equal. Try to get a good quality, especially one with a great amount of this strain. You can also treat with specific enzymes which coat the stomach lining and heal it from the inside out. See TIP #142.

TIP #156:

I love all products from Boiron. They are homeopathic products with different strengths and the bottles show the condition you want treated. The smaller the number, the stronger the product.

TIP #157:

Andrographis is a plant endemic to India. It is frequently used in combination with Siberian ginseng to prevent common colds and flu when taken during the first 3 days of the onset. It usually takes up to 5 days before most symptoms disappear. See TIPS #74, #148, #176, and #211.

TIP #158:

Masaru Emoto (1943-2014) was a researcher and photographer who was able to take pictures of water crystals and proved that when treated with aromatic oils, kind spoken or typed words after the water was crystallized, the crystals had a majestic response: clear, well-formed and visually pleasing. On the other hand, negative intentions would render odd unevenly formed blurred crystals. Words and intent do have an impact in our lives. Research him! We need to be aware of what we say and what we think. At the end, it is all about energy.

TIP #159:

For eyelash growth I add a capsule of biotin to my eyelash cream and mix it well. I use this ointment on the tip of my eyelashes. See TIP #154.

TIP #160:

Five steps to aid digestion:
- **First things first. Breathe and try to relax.**
- **Eat some bitters right before you eat. This will spark the digestive juices.**
- **Take a digestive enzyme to help you break down what your body is unable to.**
- **Eat enough good oils to aid with biliary function.**
- **And extremely important: Chew each bite at least 25 to 30 times. See TIPS #106, #207, and #319.**

TIP #161:

When you shower let clean water pour in your ears to soften the wax. Do not EVER use q-tips. Towel dry the outside of the ear only.

TIP #162:

Vitamin A:
Important for vision and immune system. The best source is sweet potato; other sources are pasture-raised beef, organic

spinach, wild-caught fish, organic eggs, carrots. See TIP #175.

TIP #163:

Vitamin B1 (thiamine):
Important to process carbohydrates. A good source is beans. See TIP #175.

TIP #164:

Vitamin B2 (riboflavin):
Helps the body make red blood cells. Good sources are asparagus, almonds, organic chicken. See TIP #175.

TIP #165:

Vitamin B3 (niacin):
Helps make cholesterol and digest food into energy. Good sources are wild-caught fish, organic chicken, pasture-raised beef, organic turkey. See TIP #175.

TIP #166:

Vitamin B5 (pantothenic acid):
You can find it in organic chicken, pasture-raised beef, organic tomatoes, and organic potatoes. It helps turn food into energy. See TIP #175.

TIP #167:

Vitamin B6:
Important for your nervous system and it helps the body break down proteins. A good source is chickpeas. Other sources are pasture-raised beef, wild-caught fish, organic baked potatoes with skin, organic eggs, organic spinach, bananas, organic turkey. See TIP #175.

TIP #168:

Vitamin B7 (Biotin):
Helps nourish cells. Good sources are organic fruits and pasture-raised meats. See TIP #175.

TIP #169:

Vitamin B12:
Helps make red blood cells. Good sources are wild-caught salmon, pasture-raised beef, wild-caught tuna, organic poultry. See TIP #175.

TIP #170:

Vitamin C:
It is one of the most important vitamins because it is involved in many biochemical procedures in the body. It boosts your immune system and it makes collagen too. A great source is organic sweet red bell peppers. Other good sources are citrus fruits, organic green bell peppers, cabbage, and organic spinach. If you are to acquire vitamin 'C' off-the-counter, purchase rose hips - a complete form of vitamin 'C'. Ascorbic acid is just one part of the vitamin rendering it incomplete. See TIP #175.

TIP #171:

Vitamin D:
Vitamin D is very important. I recommend testing your vitamin D levels every 3 months to see if you are getting enough. Vitamin D is crucial for thyroid function, a fantastic anti-oxidant, and great for the bones among other things. Make sure it does not have any fillers, especially in the capsule. Vitamin D should NOT be taken for long periods of time. Ten minutes of sun a day is usually enough to maintain normal vitamin D levels for some individuals.
It is important for bone health (calcium) paired with magnesium so it can be absorbed properly. Food sources are organic eggs, wild-caught salmon. See TIP #175.

TIP #172:

Vitamin E:
It is a great antioxidant. Great sources are sunflower seeds, almonds and organic leafy green vegetables. See TIP #175.

TIP #173:

Vitamin K:
Helps maintain bone health. Great sources are broccoli, organic kale, organic parsley, cabbage, avocado, organic grapes, kiwis. See TIP #175.

TIP #174:

Improve the muscles around your mouth. Put some cream on before you perform the following exercises:
1 - Opening your mouth as wide as possible, repeat the vowels very slowly exaggerating the movements. Repeat 20 to 30 times.

2 - Move your mouth to the right and then to the left. 20 to 30 repetitions.
3 - Stretch your mouth to both sides and hold for 20 to 30 seconds. Do 10 repetitions.

TIP #175:

Many of us take vitamins but we forget about the minerals. Mineral absorption is an issue in many parts of the world because of agricultural processes which have depleted our soil from these valuable elements in our diet; we need to replace them. I take a liquid form version of both vitamins and minerals called 'Rush.' I take it every six months or so. I do not ingest it on a daily basis but the frequency vastly depends on your eating habits. If you eat a lot of packaged, canned, processed or fast food, you really need to take it daily. See TIPS #162-173, #183-194, #179, and #180.

TIP #176:

For a mild cold, put thyme oil on the bottom of your feet and on the palm of your hands, drink hot tea (see TIP #74, bullet #3), and smell eucalyptus. Do all this right before you lie down to bed and cover up; you will start sweating. See TIPS #74, #148, #157, and #211.

TIP #177:

Heart Math is a science-based technology with 26+ years of research. By using this technology you can experience a more balanced life and reduce stress in your life as well; you will be more in control of your emotions instead of allowing your emotions to run your day. You will be able to switch from frustration to appreciation in minutes, and your productivity will improve. The best part of this technology is that it only takes 10 minutes or so, every time you do it. You can access it directly from your smart phone through an app. I bought it many years ago so I have their gadget. Either way, it works.

TIP #178:

Ghrelin (also known as lenomorelin) is a hunger-related hormone which peaks at around 1:00 pm and starts declining around 4:00 pm. Leptin is related to the feeling of satiety, energy intake and expenditure, so it is low during the day and it starts increasing at around 4:00 pm. This is a pattern we need to respect for our bodies to work in sync with the circadian cycle, otherwise we are working against our natural metabolic rhythms. Avoiding food two to three hours before sleep time will help manage your appetite. Skipping any meal goes against this concept too - you would be at risk for insulin resistance and obesity. Under this premise, dinner should be lighter than lunch.

TIP #179:

"Cell Salts" are very important because minerals are the foundation for enzyme activity and we have rapidly depleted our soils from minerals because of bad farming techniques. They come in the form of pellets. See TIPS #175 and #180.

TIP #180:

If you are not sure what mineral your body needs, you can purchase a liquid mineral test kit. The brand I like is MTK from BodyBio. All you have to do is drink it and see how your taste buds react. Does it taste bitter, sour, sweet, or salty? Your body will let you know which mineral you need by following your taste buds; if you like it, you need it. It is that simple. See TIPS #175 and #179.

TIP #181:

Many people think that soya is a good source of food. 80% of all soya is irradiated rendering it unhealthful. It especially affects girls at an early age because they can start ovulating before puberty. I eat soya but it ALWAYS has to be **100% certified organic.**

TIP #182:

Do you suffer from leg cramps? What time of day do you get them? After exercising or while sleeping? Cramps are one of the mediums your body uses for you to pay attention! If you get cramps at night or at rest, you need magnesium. If you get them after exercising, you need calcium. If you get night-time bed cramps, you might try to drink water at bed time too.

TIP #183:

Calcium:
Strengthens yours bones and helps with muscle contraction. Great sources are organic kale, organic eggs, seeds (specially sesame: 1/2 cup has 350 mg), sardines, wild-caught salmon, beans (160 mg for 1/2 cup), lentils, dried figs, and almonds. See TIP #175.

TIP #184:

Chromium:
Controls sugar in your blood. Great sources are broccoli, potatoes, fish (wild-caught), and poultry (organic.) See TIP #175.

TIP #185:

Copper:
Helps process iron. Good sources are wild-caught seafood, nuts, and seeds. See TIP #175.

TIP #186:

Folate:
Promotes heart health. Good sources are lentils, garbanzos, and dark leafy greens. See TIP #175.

TIP #187:

Iodine:
Supports your thyroid. Great sources are wild-caught seafood and seaweed. See TIP #175 and #281.

TIP #188:

Iron:
Is needed for red blood cells. Great sources are beans, lentils, organic spinach, pasture-raised beef, and organic turkey. See TIP #175.

TIP #189:

Magnesium:
Helps your muscle spasms and supports your heart. Great sources are green leafy organic vegetables, quinoa, and nuts. See TIP #175.

TIP #190:

Manganese:
Supports bone health. Good sources are nuts, beans, and other legumes. See TIP #175.

TIP #191:

Phosphorus:
Is needed for bone health and it makes energy. Good sources are peas, pasture-raised meat, and eggs. See TIP #175.

TIP #192:

Potassium:
Controls blood pressure. Great sources are yogurt, bananas, potatoes, wild-caught tuna, organic fruits and organic vegetables. See TIP #175.

TIP #193:

Selenium:
Helps manage your thyroid and protects from free radicals. Good sources are wild-caught seafood, and Brazil nuts. See TIP #175.

TIP #194:

Zinc:
Helps maintain a sense of smell and supports the immune system. Great foods are oysters, pasture-raised beef, organic spinach, pumpkin seeds, nuts, beans, and mushrooms. See TIP #175.

TIP #195:

I use a mouth guard every night to protect my teeth. You can either purchase one over-the-counter or have one done professionally by a dentist. I do not suffer from TMJ nor do I grind my teeth; I use it merely as a preventative measure.

TIP #196:

One thing you need to know about baking soda is that it contains aluminum so purchase baking soda without this metal. One of its uses is as an odor eliminator: Add baking soda to a plastic container; puncture the lid and close the container. Voilâ! You just made a natural odor eliminator without the harmful effects of chemicals.

TIP #197:

Charcoal is another great odor eliminator. Just buy tablets and place them wherever you need the smell to be absorbed. And it is also good if you feel bloated; just take an activated charcoal tablet. This feeling of bloating is related to digestive issues and lack of enzymes.

TIP #198:

Ideas to add fragrance to your house without the chemical
exposure:
Add citrus wedges to water on plates throughout the house.
Use spices such as cinnamon and nutmeg.
Add essential oils to dry flowers.

TIP #199:

Sodium Nitrate and Sodium Nitrite are preservatives used in
several processed meats such as deli meats and hot dogs.
Sodium Nitrate is linked with certain types of cancer and
Sodium Nitrite is toxic but they still use it because it gives
that bright red color to processed meat. This is one more
reason to try to buy pasture-raised meats, and if possible,
organic too. See TIP #287.

TIP #200:

**It is important to remember that 75% of our body is
water. So hydrate, hydrate, hydrate. Remember: you
should drink 1/2 your weight in ounces of PURE WATER
throughout the day (for every 10 kilograms drink 1/3 litre
of water.) Over 70% of the population is visual, so
something that works for me is filling out the jugs of
water I need to drink throughout the day. We need to
learn to drink pure water without any flavoring. See
TIPS #3, #4, and #377.**

TIP #201:

Some home treatments for Psoriasis:
Itchiness - Rub with lavender, rose or chamomile essential
                    oils

Dry Skin - Rub with wet oat meal to detach dead skin; mix
              olive and oregano oils and rub
Inflammation and Redness - Rub with calendula cream
Controlling It - Chamomile, lemon, or lavender teas

TIP #202:

Your mouthwash and toothpaste should not contain Fluoride.
Fluoride does not prevent tooth decay and it affects your IQ
among other things. Check out Attorney Michael Connett.
He is the attorney to Fluoride Action Network (FAN). He
gives us 10 top reasons why people should not use fluoride.
See TIPS #8, #60, and #82.

TIP #203:

There is a difference between a high-speed and a low-speed
juicer. High-speed juicers oxidize the ingredients, and by
that I mean, it lets oxygen get in and the nutritional qualities
change. When you use a high speed device, drink the
concoction as soon as possible. See TIP #12.

TIP #204:

Cows are bred to give milk. They are unable to produce the
amount of milk required of them so they are injected
hormones and fed artificially so they can grow faster. All
those hormones come through the milk. If you are to drink
cow milk, make sure it comes from cows who have been
raised on green pastures and with no added antibiotics. See
TIP #24.

TIP #205:

All foods have either an alkaline effect or an acidic effect in our bodies. When we eat foods that have an acidic effect our body will experience poor digestion. In general, alkaline forming foods are foods that come from Mother Earth: Most fresh uncooked fruits, green raw leafy vegetables, green vegetables, lentils, beans, herbs, seeds and some nuts. Foods that have an acidic effect will fall in the following categories: wheat, dairy, corn, red and white potatoes, peanuts, pork, red meat, ALL processed foods. As you can see, in general, we eat acidic foods excessively and this is one of the basic causes of disease especially arthritic or rheumatic related diseases. Not everyone needs the same types of foods. Check your pH daily so you can manage your eating habits. Several stores sell pH kits with instructions on how to use them. Your pH should range between 6.5 and 7. See TIP #105.

TIP #206:

Two tablespoons of chia seeds contain fiber, high-quality protein, fat, calcium, manganese, magnesium, and phosphorus. This small serving will give you only one gram of carbohydrates and 137 calories. Fiber does not raise blood sugar so it should not be counted as carbs. Chia seeds are loaded with antioxidants and are good for bone-health since they are high in protein, calcium, magnesium, and phosphorus which are good for bones. See TIPS # 87 and #100.

TIP #207:

Enzymes: My favorite subject!
Enzymes are a part of life. They are involved in every single biochemical reaction in our bodies. According to

the #1 eminence in enzyme nutrition, Dr. Howard Loomis:

"Enzyme nutrition is the art and science of using nutrition to maintain homeostasis and health in the body. It works with the body's innate intelligence to bring the body to optimal health using whole foods that contain protein, carbohydrates, fats, vitamins, minerals, and enzymes, rather than trying to manipulate it by using chemical compounds that produce side effects. When you use enzymes you should expect:

> A decrease in gastric complaints
> A change in your bowel routine
> Increase in energy level
> Improved sleep
> Improved hormone balance
> Decreased pain and inflammation
> Decreased stored weight
> A change in appetite and food cravings
> Slowed or reversed symptoms of aging."

See TIPS #49, 54, #106, #142, #155, #160, #219, #222, #276, #310, #319, #320, and #346.

TIP #208:

Remember that you and your entire family breathe in the products you use to clean your home. Beware of ammonia, antibacterial cleaners, bleach, laundry soap, oven cleaners, plug-ins, etc. Nothing with scents, fragrance, etc. Some brands I use: Method, Mrs. Meyer's, Seventh Generation, Green Rebel, and plenty more. Or make your own; there are many recipes on the internet available to us. See TIP #39.

TIP #209:

We need to realize that there are more than 90,000 chemicals bombarding our food supply and, according to the National Research Council, there is no toxic information available for more than 80% of them. So rethink what you use. We will never get rid of all chemicals, but the less we utilize, the healthier our life will be. For example: people can have hidden sensitivities to bromine in bread or chlorine in water. <u>Are you poisoning your family?</u> Check Chem Conscious.

TIP #210:

A civil and environmental engineer by the name of Professor Steinemman from the University of Washington investigated Plug-ins and discovered they are loaded with VOCs (volatile organic compounds) which have negative health effects on your nose, eyes, and throat; you can also experience nausea, headaches, and it can damage your kidneys and liver. Use diffused oils instead.

TIP #211:

Nasal Saline Wash is fantastic for allergies and for keeping your nose clean. Always use distilled water or boil water and let it cool to room temperature. Lean forward and let half of the saline water go in through one nostril and out the other; then switch sides and finish the rest of the saline water. Blow your nose gently. See TIPS #74, #132, #144, #148, #157, #176, and #215.

TIP #212:

Here are some ideas on how to prepare four nutritious meals in less than 20 minutes (taken from Dr. Christianson's web page):

(Italics represent my insertions or comments)
Bowls
Salads
Soups
Stir-frys

Veggies:
All veggies should be organic (see TIP #20 and #21)
Spinach
Chopped onions
Grape/cherry tomatoes
Chopped/shredded cabbage
Chopped/shredded carrots
Broccoli heads
Sliced mushrooms
And most other veggies are fairly quick to chop when you need them.

Protein:
Certified organic meat, chopped: beef, chicken, turkey
Canned sardines
I intentionally omitted the other options. I do not believe canned chicken or deli meat such as ham are healthful for you.

Carbs:
Beans (heat on stove). Beans are a great source of protein too. *See TIP #69.*
Cooked beets
Lentils
Hummus
Sweet potatoes (frozen) shredded

Boiled potatoes (once water boils, it takes 9 minutes to cook).

When using carbs, do not use meats in the same dish. Use one or the other.

Healthful fats:
Extra-virgin olive oil (*use only cold for salads or other dishes*)
Avocado
Avocado or coconut oils (to cook)
Almonds (*always soak overnight before using*) *(See TIP #56).*
Cashews, macadamias, walnuts, pecans
Olives
Seeds

Toppings:
Cilantro *(organic)*
Parsley *(organic)*
Ginger
Lime/lemon
Garlic
Chopped tomatoes *(organic)*
Epazote

TIP #213:

Breakfast bars:
Energy bars are very tricky. The majority of them are loaded with sugar or artificial sweeteners; and even if they have good-quality sweeteners they are loaded with sugar, and we need to avoid as much sugar as possible. I have found three different bars which only have 1, 4, and 6 grams of plant-sourced sugar respectively: Unstoppable Bar (from Dr. Ritamarie Loscalzo), Know Cow, and Sun Warrior, all of them are high-protein bars. If you choose to experiment, try sprouted grain bars from Sun Warrior or Go Raw.

TIP #214:

The best tips to move your bowels are: drink a lot of water, exercise, and eat fiber. One awesome fruit to help you have a bowel movement is prunes. Just eat 4 to 6 prunes and that will do the trick. If you still haven't had a bowel movement, take a bit more; but go slowly if you don't want to be surprised.

TIP #215:

Propolis is a sticky substance from the trees which bees carry to their hive to seal holes and to entirely varnish it. During the XIX and XX centuries it was used as a natural antibiotic. Since 1970, it has been found that it has great fungicidal and bactericidal properties. It is great for skin diseases such as eczema, psoriasis, light burns, scratches, acne, boils, etc. It has been found good to prevent colds, laryngitis, pharyngitis, sinusitis, bronchitis, etc. Beware: Some people are allergic to bee products. I take it during cold season which, for me, is from October through March. See TIP #144.

TIP #216:

Golden Paste:
Use organic turmeric powder. Turmeric stains so be very careful.
In a pan at medium-low setting, heat 1/2 cup water with 1/4 cup turmeric and continually stir for 7 to 9 minutes. If it starts drying out, add more water until you get a medium consistency. Put the paste in a glass container and wait until it cools down to put it in the refrigerator. It will last up to14 to 21 days. Use it to make Golden Milk. Compliments of Ayurvedic Medicine. SEE TIPS #30 and # 217.

TIP #217:

Golden Milk:
1/2 teaspoon of turmeric paste (TIP #216)
1 cup unsweetened milk (organic cow, 100% organic soya, almond, hemp, etc.)
Warm up in a pot. Then add:
1/4 tsp almond oil, sesame oil, or Udos oil
(Good oils help lubricate the joints.)
1/8 tsp raw honey or maple syrup
If someone has severe pain, they can take 1/2 teaspoon to 1 teaspoon twice a day. See TIP #30.

TIP #218:

Beta-Sitosterol together with Niacin No-Flush is a great way to lower cholesterol combined with exercise and a healthful diet. Take them as directed on the bottle. Always check with your physician first. This was given to me by a very dear friend and holistic doctor based in Huntington Park, CA, Dr. Luis Muñoz.

TIP #219:

Have you ever thought why people either make too much saliva and spit everywhere or not enough. If you make too much saliva you might have issues digesting protein and your jaw might be tight too. If you have a dry mouth, you might have issues digesting carbohydrates. Solution: Digestive enzymes for those specific categories. See TIP #340.

TIP #220:

Celery is an excellent source of fiber, helps avoid water
retention (PMS), and helps with the stomach lining. Eat
three or four pieces with humus, raw organic nut butters,
good quality cheese (if not allergic to dairy and cannot live
without cheese), pico de gallo, etc.

TIP #221:

In order to know how many grams of protein you need on a
daily basis, follow this formula:
Your body weight in pounds times 0.9 divided by 2.2 = daily
grams of protein.
Your body weight in kilograms times 0.9 = daily grams of
protein.

TIP #222:

Problems falling asleep:
Hot bath with epsom salts and take enzymes, melatonin, or
valerian root to help you sleep. Always check with your
doctor when taking supplements.

TIP #223:

Beef, pork, and poultry are fed hormones so they can get
fatter and grow faster with a minimum amount of space to
move around in their own excrement. Their living conditions
are undesirable and stressful. Chicken, turkeys, and pigs
are thrown in trucks, alive, piled one on top of the other and
go through horrendous inhumane processes to get to your
plate. We need to be more conscious, not only for the
animals but also for us. We are eating all the hormones,
antibiotics, and adrenaline secreted by these poor creatures.

We need to buy humane, certified, organic, pasture-raised, free-range beef, pork, and poultry so they can have a decent life and we can ingest decent food free of all those additions which our body is unable to process, and we will be helping our planet on the way: It takes inordinate amounts of energy to produce meat.

TIP #224:

If you eat out, ask questions:
1 - Ask what type of fish you are eating; there are several fish which are created hydroponically; try to eat wild-caught fish instead.
2 - Order your food with no sauces, they are loaded with sugar and salt.
3 - Order your food with no added salt.
4 - Order vegetables and grilled protein.
The closest to Mother Earth's natural process of creation, the healthier we will be.

TIP #225:

**Organic vs Conventional. Many individuals do not see the need to pay a higher price for organically grown products versus conventionally grown ones.
Organically grown products cost more because producers have to prove that their products do not use "added ingredients" such as insecticides, pesticides, herbicides, antibiotics, dyes, artificial sweeteners, etc. which conventionally grown products are loaded with. Some of these "added ingredients" used in the United States have been banned in developed countries throughout the world. See TIPS #20, #21, #76, #241 and #306.**

TIP #226:

According to Leo Heart, our cells listen to what we say and perceive what we feel. This is part of a science called PsychoNeuroImmunology (PNI) which studies the interaction among the chemical processes, the nervous system, the immune system, and the endocrine system of the human body. That is why we need to be very aware, not only of what we say, but also of what we think and what we feel because that has an impact on our health.

TIP # 227:

Cut limes in half and insert several pieces of clove half way so as to keeping them from falling. Do these with several limes and place them around your environment. It deters mosquitoes! See TIPS #121, #255, #360, and #367.

TIP #228:

Flaxseeds are a great antioxidant and they have a great amount of soluble and insoluble fiber, as well as lowering cholesterol. Buy them whole and keep them tight and in a dark container. Grind them as you use them; don't buy ground flaxseed. Be cautious - they might cause bowel obstruction in large dosis. Daily amount: one tablespoon in a food processor and then sprinkle on food or in water, smoothie, juice, yoghurt, etc.

TIP #229:

Water and heart attacks. A friend of mine told me her doctor recommended the following:
2 glasses of water upon awakening - helps activate internal organs.

1 glass of water before meals - helps with digestion.
1 glass of water before taking a shower - will lower your blood pressure.
1 glass of water before going to bed - may avoid a stroke or a heart attack.
If nothing else, water will NOT hurt you.

TIP #230:

God's Food nourishes different parts of your body:

Carrots, when seen sliced, have the shape of an eye
Celery has the shape of a bone
Grapefruit has the shape of a mammary gland
Grapes, in clusters, have the shape of a heart
Tomatoes, when sliced, have the shape of a heart; they have 4 chambers
Walnuts have the shape of a small brain.

ENJOY!

TIP #231:

If you are marinating food, always use glass containers.
And remember: try to use fresh ingredients versus a bottled sauce.

TIP #232:

Stevia is a green leafy plant originated in Paraguay and been used by its indigenous habitants for millennia. In its natural state it is 20 times sweeter than sugar. Try to get a plant and use it in salads or dry it and grind it and use it instead of processed sugar. If you are going to buy some, it needs to be green in color and stevia as the only ingredient.

Check "Dulce Revolución" which stands for Sweet Revolution, European site. I have seen several brands advertise stevia as "natural", "raw", "organic", etc., etc., etc., and when you read the ingredients the first one is sugar disguised under a different name. BEWARE!!! See TIP #35.

TIP #233:

If you love gardening or are committed to growing your food supply, High Mowing Seed Company is a great source of 100% organic seeds. See TIP #260.

TIP #234:

Your body is a wonderful and superb machine; it knows exactly what to do to keep you alive. When we condemn certain parts of our body we are disrupting the energy that was so perfectly created. We need to accept and love our bodies the way they are RIGHT NOW in order to heal emotionally and move forward. One great exercise is to stand in front of a long mirror where you can see your body from head to toe and completely nude. Starting from top to bottom and in descending order, give thanks to each internal and external part of your body and to all the systems as well; try to be as detailed as possible:
Thank you head
Thank you hair
Thank you brain
Thank you skull
Thank you neurological system
Thank you forehead, etc.
Pay attention to which organ or system you skip or what you forget; it might need attention.

TIP #235:

Every morning upon awakening give thanks for 3 things; it sets the mood for the rest of the day. And every night at bed time give thanks for 3 different things. Try to find different things to be thankful for each time you do it. It changes the way you see life and you will feel better. Guaranteed!!

TIP #236:

Our digestion starts the moment we start thinking about food. Choosing healthful foods is one part of the digestion process but it is not the only one. There are two more important parts: Environment and chewing. We need to be calm to digest food: Blessing your food and/or deep breathing will help with that part. And the last one is chewing: We need to chew each bite at least 20 to 30 times.

TIP #237:

Difference among Suntan Lotion, Sunscreen, and Sunblock:
Suntan Lotion will not protect you from the sun rays. It usually has oils which do not protect you from the sun.
Sunscreen will protect you from the ultraviolet rays letting some go through.
Sunblock will not allow any rays penetrate the skin.
My choice: Sunblock.

TIP #238:

Want to improve your jaw line:
1 - Try to touch your tongue to your palate throughout the day.

2 - Place your hand in front of your forehead applying pressure while you push your head forward. Count to 30 slowly.

3 - Place your hand on the back of your head applying pressure while you push your head back. Count to 30 slowly.

4 - Place your hand on the left side of your head applying pressure while you push your head to the left. Count to 30 slowly.

5 - Repeat with the right side.

TIP #239:

When standing, we need to be conscious of our posture. If we slouch we are adding undo pressure to our internal organs and we are unable to oxygenate our body properly.

- **Stand up straight pulling your shoulders back and down. We instinctively move them up and down, but it should be BACK and down.**
- **Set your feet straight and put weight on the outer part of your feet and on the ball of your feet. And try to raise your toes.**
- **Pull your stomach in and up.**

TIP #240:

When sitting push your buttocks all the way to the back of the seat. This will give your upper back more support. Move your shoulders back and down. We tend to move them up and down but the movement should be BACK and down.

TIP #241:

GMO stands for Genetically Modified Organisms. GMO food is food which has being altered genetically by manipulating the structure of cells not only by adding to or taking away from, but also by transferring from one organism to another across species. These foods are created in a lab so I do not consider them food. Foods that are made with corn, canola or soy usually contain GMOs. "Consumer Reports" is a more reliable and neutral source to learn more about it. GMO labeling has been made mandatory in more than 60 countries throughout the world but not in the United States. By the way, GMOs are not only in fruit and vegetables; they are found in all sorts of packaged food such as cereals, snacks, breads, etc. See TIPS #20, #21, #76, #225, and #306.

TIP #242:

If you have a headache squeeze the web between the thumb and the index fingers for several minutes until it subsides. See TIP #149.

TIP #243:

Since millennia natives have utilized charcoal to clean their teeth. Burn a corn tortilla and pulverize it; this is truly activated charcoal. See TIP #248.

TIP # 244:

Baby colic: Use charcoal on TIP #243 and add a pinch to baby's milk.

TIP #245:

Processed sugar lowers testosterone by 20%. We need testosterone to build muscle. See TIPS #5 and #35.

TIP #246:

If you are a woman and wake up between 2:00 am and 4:00 am, you might need progesterone cream. Check with your primary care doctor.

TIP #247:

If you love ice cream, try to find one which has no colorings (violet, blue, red, yellow, green.....), additives, artificial preservatives, etc. There are a couple of descent brands called Talenti and Halo Top. I do not eat ice cream because almost all of them have processed sugar and I do not drink cow's milk either, but, in my opinion, these are decent brands.

TIP #248:

I use a mineral powder or activated charcoal to whiten my teeth by the name of Geopharm (from Mexico). No preservatives, no pain, no sensitivity. Just minerals. It will not whiten your teeth overnight but with continuous use, it will. See TIP #243.

TIP #249:

For lots of women out there: Even though your numbers might be within "normal range" regarding hypothyroidism, you might still be experiencing symptoms such as low energy, loss of hair (clumps), difficulty losing weight, high cholesterol, dry skin, cold hands and feet, and constipation among others. Hypothyroidism can also present itself through carpal tunnel, joint pain, shoulder pain, edema, and inflammation. Measuring your T-3 is not enough. They need to measure your antibodies and if they are within normal range, then order a complete panel: T-3, T-4, reverse T-3, and reverse T-4. Some individuals cannot convert T4 to T3. See TIPS #92, #187, #193, #257, #281, #342, #345, and #352.

TIP #250:

I use vitamin 'E' oil on each nail and toenail to keep them lubricated. I do this just before I leave the house so they look nice and shiny. See TIPS #44, #45, and #317.

TIP #251:

We usually carry our handbag on the same shoulder day in and day out. This is not good for our bone structure. If we continue with this pattern, eventually our body will be misaligned. Switch sides every so often.

TIP #252:

Fit Brain and Lumosity are two great websites to exercise your brain.

TIP #253:

Rosemary has fantastic properties. It is a well rounded herb which contains vitamins 'A' and 'C', and high in calcium, potassium, iron, magnesium, salt, zinc, and phosphorus. Boil it and take it as tea. Or cook with it too.

TIP #254:

Parsley is a great diuretic. Boil it, let it cool down, and drink the water throughout the day.

TIP #255:

A friend of mine sent me this information:
Homemade Mosquito Trap:
1 cup of water
1/4 cup of brown sugar
1 gram of yeast
1 2-litre bottle

- Cut plastic bottle in half
- Mix brown sugar with hot water. Let cool. When cold, pour it in the bottom half of the bottle
- Add the yeast. No need to mix. It creates carbon dioxide which attracts mosquitoes
- Place the funnel part, upside down, into the other half of the bottle, taping them together if desired
- Wrap the bottle with something black, leaving the top uncovered, and place it outside in an area away from your normal gathering area
- CHANGE the solution every two weeks for continuous control. See TIPS #121, #227, and #360, and #367.

TIP #256:

Chromium Polinicotinate is a great supplement to level sugar in the blood. This might benefit you if you are diabetic (ask your doctor first). If you are eating something sweet, take one capsule with your meal. WATCH OUT: Polinicotinate and not picolinate.

TIP #257:

Great supporters for the thyroid are: ashwagandha, cordyceps, and brazil nuts. Use them in your smoothies. See TIPS #92, #100, #187, #193, #249, #281, #342, #345, and #352.

TIP #258:

Have you heard of kinesiology taping? It is a rehabilitative technique to support and stabilize injured muscles or joints by facilitating the body's natural healing process. According to "Kinesiotaping", the tape is "......**specifically applied** to the patient based upon their needs after evaluation." Very well accepted among athletes: KT Tape.

TIP #259:

Do you want to learn if something is good for your body or not? This is known as muscle testing:
You need a partner.
Grab something you want tested; this could be anything from a packet of sugar to a book; the sky is the limit.
- Stand straight ahead and face each other.
- Grab what you want tested in one hand and raise the other hand to one side so it is parallel to the floor at shoulder level.
- Look straight into the wall right in front of you. Do not look at your partner, just straight to the wall in front of you.
- Ask your partner to put slight pressure on the wrist of the raised arm and ask him/her to push down.
- Don't resist; just let your body react.

If your arm comes down easily with very little resistance, whatever object you are holding is not good for you.

TIP #260:
If you are a gardener or would like to become one, two great places which sell 100% Certified Organic seeds are "Annie's Heirloom Seeds" and "Seeds of Change". See TIP #233.

TIP #261:

Buying nuts, superfoods, and seeds which are non-GMO. may be expensive. Frontier Coop is a great source. You can purchase great things, sometimes in bulk, at much lower prices. See TIP #262.

TIP #262:

I know that getting organic, non-GMO veggies and fruits may be expensive. With the use of the internet there are more avenues accessible to all of us. We have CSAs (Community Supported Agriculture) which, like their name suggests, they are an easier and less expensive way for consumers to buy local, seasonal food directly from the farmer. Check their website to find a CSA close to you: localharvest.org. There is also another link called ImperfectProduce.com which will sell organic imperfect produce at a lower price. See TIP #261.

TIP #263:

Bach Flowers are fantastic for managing emotions. You can find them in different stores or on line, and they have zero side effects. If your are interested in taking it a step further, there are many Certified Natural Health Professionals that can evaluate you.

TIP #264:

Ears, palms of hands, and bottom of feet are a map to your body parts. If you make a habit of rubbing them, with love and patience, you will be massaging all your body. Pay attention to which points hurt, and investigate what organs they represent and work on them by massaging them constantly and by eating properly.

TIP #265:

There is a great book by Louise Hay which is called: "Heal Your Mind, Heal Your Body." It is replete with affirmations supporting each organ/system of your body. I am a firm believer that health is not only physical; it is a compilation of emotions, thoughts, genes, and diet.

TIP #266:

Your food can impact not only your body but also your feelings. A simple way to test for allergies or sensitivities: Check your pulse before and after you eat. A raise of 10 points might show an indication of allergy.
Check your feelings 8 to 24 hours after you eat something. Crummy feelings???? Crummy feelings equate to Crummy Food!!!! Remember we are all not made the same so some things might not affect you and they might affect someone else. See TIPS #98, 141, and #314.

TIP #267:

Table Salt increases blood pressure. Is there a need to say more.... See TIP #96.

TIP #268:

Good cookware brands: All-Clad, Calphalon, Hestan NanoBond, etc. Just make sure it has no teflon or sticky surface and that they are made of stainless steel. See TIPS #63, #65 and #66.

TIP #269:

Water is very important for our bodies AND we need to know what's in it. There are many testing kits you can purchase to do so. In my opinion, we all need to have a 'reverse osmosis' system or make sure you use some sort of carbon filter. If you cannot have a home system, the least you need to do is place a filter in your shower head and one in your kitchen faucet. The system I have at home is from Sweet Water.

TIP #270:

Nutritional Yeast is a great source of dietary fiber, it is excellent for brain cells.   It is an excellent complement to legumes. You can also use it as a cheese substitute.

TIP #271:

Raw dieters as well as seniors need to take B12. On average, 1,000 micrograms per day may be best.

TIP #272:

Leafy Greens and green vegetables are very rich in calcium and folate. They protect your blood vessels and are nutrient-dense. See TIP #100 to introduce them to your diet in an easy way. Or just use them in salads.

TIP #273:

Recipe for alkaline water:
In one gallon of distilled water, add one teaspoon of calcium powder, one teaspoon of aluminum-free baking soda, and the juice of one lime. Stir well and leave in refrigerator.

TIP #274:

Here are some herbs and spices that alkalize. Disease does not thrive in an alkaline environment but it does in an acidic one:
Cardamom, cilantro, cinnamon, ginger, peppermint, turmeric. Use them in smoothies, sprinkle them over food, and cook with them too.

TIP #275:

According to Jin Shin Jyutsu you can balance your emotions by holding your fingers. Each one is linked to an emotion:

Thumb	represents	**Worry, stress, tension**
Index finger	represents	**Fear**
Middle finger	represents	**Anger, frustration, indecision**
Ring finger	represents	**Sadness, grief**
Little finger	represents	**Pretense**

All you have to do is wrap one finger with your other hand for two to five minutes or as long you need to until you feel a pulse; then proceed to the next finger. Do this with both hands.

TIP #276:

Want to ward off neurological diseases:
Multivitamin, antioxidant complex, macro-mineral complex,
probiotics, and food enzymes with every meal. B vitamins to
support the nervous system.   See TIP #383.

TIP #277:

Red clover helps with cough. If you are using the herb itself
use 2 tsp of the dried flowers in 8 oz (240 ml) of hot water for
45 minutes and drink 3 to 4 cups every day.
Another great mix is honey and cinnamon in equal amounts;
make a paste and take a teaspoon every so often to soothe
the coughing.

TIP #278:

Use the following concoction to strengthen the ligaments and
knees:
2 oz (55 grams) of powdered almonds
1 oz (28 grams) of pure honey
1cup of water
1/8 tsp of cinnamon
1cup of oatmeal
2 cups of pineapple juice
2 cups of orange juice

Boil the water and add the oatmeal. Stir for 5 minutes. Add
all the other ingredients and combine.

TIP #279:

Another idea to flavor water is to make some ice cubes out of lemon juice, lime juice, orange juice, etc. Use them for tea as well: Boil water and add a cube or two to it.

TIP #280:

The healthy eating pyramid should look like this: At the base should be Water, then Greens, then Fruit, then legumes, then herbs, and, at the end, any meat/ dairy.

TIP #281:

Some foods that boost your thyroid are wild-caught salmon, brazil nuts, herring, sesame seeds, pumpkin seeds, spinach, olive oil, avocado oil, almonds, and hazelnuts. See TIPS #92, #187, #193, #249, #257, #342, #345, and #352.

TIP #282:

If you are breastfeeding and your newborn has colic your nutrition might be the cause of it. Are you eating dairy, chocolate, caffeine, raw onion, peanuts, chiles? These are all irritants.

TIP #283:

The glands around your eyes may clog for several reasons. What you can do to keep them healthy is hot compresses on your eyelids for 10 to 15 minutes a day. As hot as you can handle them without burning yourself. See TIP #284.

TIP #284:

Another way to help your glands around your eyes is when you are taking a shower, put your index finger horizontally and gently press up and then press down. See TIP #283.

TIP #285:

I heard someone once say: "Where are you when you are in the shower?" Our society is so fast-paced we do not allow ourselves to experience the moment. This is a huge CHALLENGE for many of us. We are doing something and thinking on what's next. We miss so much by living this way. I challenge you and your brain: BE PRESENT! When you are doing something FOCUS 100% of your attention on that one thing.

TIP #286:

If you are going to eat bread, please eat something that does not convert to sugar. No white bread, white flour, flour tortillas, crackers, etc. The best thing you can do is to buy grain-based bread or gluten-free (if you cannot live without bread). I love "Know Better" which is an organic, non-GMO, nut-based bread. Another brand I choose is Ezequiel; it is a wheat-based bread which has been processed differently. See TIP #49.

TIP #287:

Dirty dozen food additives that should be avoided:

Nitrites and Nitrates
Potassium Bromate
Propyl Paraben

Butylated Hydroxianisole (BHA)
Butylated Hydroxytoluene (BHT)
Propyl Gallate
Theobromine
Flavor Ingredients
Artificial Colors
Diacetyl
Phosphate Food Additives
Aluminum Additives
(Courtesy of EWG) See TIPS #111, #114, #115, #199, #300, and #357.

TIP #288:

Cut a pear or an apple in small pieces. Boil it with a small amount of water (just enough for it not to stick.) Mash the fruit, add chopped nuts to it and mix well. If you need to sweeten it, try raw honey or lucuma powder. Enjoy!

TIP #289:

Magnesium helps you fall asleep. Buy a good quality and mix it with water. Spray on your hands and chest or mist the air. Happy sleeping!

TIP #290:

Processed peanut butter is not very healthful; it is usually loaded with sugar and unhealthful oils. It is better to grind your own peanuts or go to the bulk section of your supermarket and grind them there. This way you will be sure there are no added ingredients. Be daring: try different butters: Cashews are sweeter, almonds are crunchier.

TIP #291:

If you are sitting for too long or use the computer, get up
every 2 to 3 hours and stretch for a couple of minutes. You
will not only destress your body but will yield more at work.
Try the following stretching exercises:
- Stand up and touch your toes 2 or 3 times.
- Turn your head to the right and count to 10.
- Turn your head to the left and count to 10.
- Grab behind your right arm with your left arm and
stretch for a count of 10.
- Grab behind your left arm with your right arm and
stretch for a count of 10.

TIP #292:

Basil is a a great alkaline herb.   It helps prevent oxidative
damage to the liver according to the Journal of American
Science in 2011. Add it to salads or soups.

TIP #293:

Red clover is very good for eczema and psoriasis. Use it in
the form of an ointment as needed. If you have an open
wound don't use it.

TIP #294:

**THERE IS NO AVERAGE PERSON. We should not have
the same parameters for a woman who is 5' (1.5 meters)
tall weighing 110 lbs (45 kilograms) versus a man who is
7' (2.10 meters) tall weighing 180 lbs (82 kilograms). It
does not make any sense. We are all individuals and we
should all be treated as such.**

TIP #295:

We need to realize that health is not only impacted by food, but also by emotions. Our bodies are energy and sometimes emotions get stuck in our bodies disallowing the energy flow. If we brew and brew and brew on past or present negative experiences, they will impact our cells and disease will set in. **Health is a combination of food, stress, genes, and emotions.** We need to deal with our emotions by expressing them and/or letting them go. Once I heard someone say: There are only two things to worry about: Those things you can change and those you cannot. If you can change them, do something about it or stop worrying if you choose not to do anything! If you cannot change them, let them go, don't worry.

TIP #296:

Stress can slow down our digestion. We need to sit down, breathe, and concentrate on eating slowly, thanking the food we are eating at that very moment. Being present is something we need to work on. Just think: "Where are you when you are in the shower?" "If you are stirring the pot, stir the pot!"

TIP #297:

Try something outside your comfort zone: On the premises that your body is pure energy, we can deduce that if we continually have a self-negative talk, we are affecting the vibrations of our surroundings and our bodies. I will share with you what I did when I was having to undergo a breast biopsy. I wrote down on a minute piece of paper the words: "I love you! Please forgive me!" I placed this piece of paper in my bra with the words facing my breast and used it every single day. No harm in doing so, right? I believe everything is energy! By the way, results came in negative.

TIP #298:

Ho'oponopono is a Hawaiian practice to reconcile and forgive. It consists of four steps: repentance, forgiveness, gratitude, and love. So if you wish to heal a situation, something or someone, just repeat over and over again: "I am sorry, forgive me, I love you, I bless you!

TIP #299:

I try to use the least amount of chemicals as possible and that includes cosmetics too. This is what I use:

Bath products:	**Epsom salts and coconut oil**
Body scrub:	**Made at home, see TIP #330**
Body lotion:	**Non-fragrant, shea butter based or coconut oil based (or just pure coconut oil once once or twice a month.)**
Body soap:	**Charcoal based**
Body wash:	**Spearmint or Lavender, see TIP #315**
Cosmetics:	**Sunshine Botanicals, Minerals**
Facial Cleanser:	**Earth Science, Clinique**
Facial Toner:	**Chamomile tea bags in water, see TIP #356**
Facial Scrub:	**Alba Botanica**
Foot & hand cream:	**Made at home, see TIP #75**
Hand Salve:	**TIP #131**
Mascara:	**Zuzu (gluten free) or Thrive Causemetics**
Veggie Cleaner:	**Rebel Green, see TIP #336**

I haven't found any products besides the above mentioned that I like to replace all the other products with. I am still searching.

TIP #300:

BHA and BHT are preservatives which you find in processed food such as potato chips, and cereals. It gives them a longer shelf-life but they are known to alter behavior. Do you have kids with personality issues? See TIP #287.

TIP #301:

I rub coconut oil on my hair and leave it on for a couple hours before showering. Try to get a raw, organic coconut oil. It should not have a liquid consistency; it should be creamy and white in color. I do this every 3 to 4 months.

TIP #302:

Robert Holden (British psychologist and writer) has an 8-week course on how to "Be Happy". It is also known as Positive Psychology. Happiness can be measured through BHI (Be Happy Index). It is a learned process and it is something anyone can acquire by using certain processes. Happiness is a choice. Let's make that choice and be happy every day no matter what we are experiencing!!! Route for yourself!! No one else knows when you need it the most!

TIP #303:

The word essential comes from the word "essence" which is extracted from the plant. If you add an oil carrier to an essence, it will last longer and will not evaporate as fast. One of the most commonly known is lavender oil which is very relaxing - use it in a diffuser at night or in a bubble bath. Juniper has a diuretic effect. Thyme helps when you have colds (on your hands and feet). Eucalyptus will help you breathe better. Tea tree is great for fighting infections.

TIP #304:

Recipe for a healthful snack:
 Vegetable Pico:
2 Carrots
1 Cup celery root or 4 celery stalks
4 Radishes
1 Red onion
1 Endive
4 Roma tomatoes (cored)
1/2 Bunch cilantro
1 1/2 Lemons (or to taste)
Sea or Himalayan salt and pepper to taste
2 Tbsp ground cumin

Add carrots, celery root (or celery stalks), red onion, radishes, and endive in food processor, chop finely, and pour in a bowl.
Chop tomatoes.
Chop cilantro finely.
Combine all ingredients and add lemon juice, salt, pepper, cumin and mix well.
Enjoy! Compliments of Moi!

TIP #305:

Fulvic acid contains a plethora of nutrients such as electrolytes, trace minerals, pre-biotics and probiotics. It is a very good product to improve your gut's good bacteria.

TIP #306:

The difference between organic and certified organic lies on the percentage of ingredients which are organic in the products you purchase.
The word ORGANIC means that animals have to be pasture-raised and not fed hormones or antibiotics; and fruits and vegetables cannot be exposed to pesticides, herbicides, fertilizers or sewage sludge.
Certified 100% organic means that 100% of the ingredients are organic.
Certified organic means that 95 to 99% of the ingredients are organic.
Organic means that 70% of the ingredients are organic. See TIPS #20, #21, #76, #225, and **#241**.

TIP #307:

Brush your teeth in the direction your gums grow. Brush your upper teeth starting at the root of the teeth toward the bottom, one stroke at a time separating the tooth brush after each stroke. Repeat the same movement with your lower teeth starting at the root of the teeth toward the top. Brush your teeth in the direction your gums grow. DO NOT brush them from side to side. Save your gums!

TIP #308:

There are many foods out there which are labeled organic which are loaded with sugar. Marketers use the word "organic" very loosely inducing people to believe that just because it says organic it is healthful and it is not. ALWAYS READ THE INGREDIENTS. **Even if it is labeled organic, if it is junk food it is still junk food, nothing changes. Junk food includes: candy, ice cream, pop corn, fried foods, energy drinks, chips, chocolate, etc.** See TIP #111.

TIP #309:

Metabolic Syndrome:
Do you crave sweets just after eating a meal?
Do you have a hard time losing weight even if you exercise?
Do you have a hard time getting rid of your mid-section fat?
Do you get fatigued mid afternoon?
Do you have high blood pressure?
Do you have high sugar levels?
Do you urinate excessively?
Metabolic Syndrome is closely linked to excess weight (obesity) and lack of activity. If you have three or more of these symptoms, you should seek help.

TIP #310:

If you suffer from acid reflux or heartburn you need to stop eating pork, onions (cooked or raw), radishes, tomatoes (of any kind), cucumbers, cabbage (raw or cooked) and absolutely nothing fried. And you need specific enzymes to build the lining of your stomach.

TIP #311:

Colorings or dyes such as yellow 6, blue 4, red 5, etc., are all additives used to make items more appealing to your eye, but they are not good for you. They cause allergies and serious illnesses to many people. You can find them in candy, meat, pet food, ice cream, medications, clothing, etc. Unless you check that the specific source comes from a fruit or a vegetable, avoid them at all cost.

TIP #312:

Bilberry is an excellent source of vitamin A and C. It helps with night vision, visual fatigue, and myopia.

TIP #313:

Relaxation is very important for healing. It is estimated that 75 to 90% of the visits to a primary care physician are related to stress (American Institute of Stress). There are many tools out there to learn to relax: meditation, deep breathing, heart math, transcendental meditation, yoga, etc. See TIPS #177 and #321.

TIP #314:

Allergy sufferers? Check your diet first and eliminate ALL processed, packaged, fast AND canned foods. Then sprinkle a mixture of turmeric, basil leaf, and coriander in your foods. See TIPS #98, #141 and #266.

TIP #315:

Spearmint is very good for refreshing the body. Lavender is very relaxing. Take a bunch of either one and insert it in a fine mesh bag; use it to scrub yourself in the shower. Spearmint also serves as a deodorant for the body, and definitely as tea. See TIP #299.

TIP #316:

Having tummy problems? Boil rue (or ruda) for about 5 minutes, let it cool to room temperature and sweeten it with some honey. This tea is great for tummy aches.

TIP #317:

Home-made nail hardener:
One clove of garlic finely chopped
Clear nail polish
Use it every night.

TIP #318:

Water has many benefits. It will obviously keep you hydrated but it will also improve digestion and help with constipation. It keeps your brain and your body energized. It may relieve headaches if it is due to dehydration.   Some of the symptoms of dehydration are: inability to sweat, headaches, confusion, lightheadedness, chills, and increased heart rate. (This happened to my dad and he ended up in the emergency room. It took him about 4 to 5 days to be able to be at his best again).

TIP #319:

As I mentioned before, enzymes is my favorite subject and my favorite supplementation to my diet. If you ever feel sluggish after a meal, if your energy is not even throughout the day, if you feel tired in the late afternoon and feel like taking a nap, if you have headaches, if you experience bloating or gas, if you lack sleep or experience insomnia, if you cannot fall asleep easily, if you have warts, etc., etc. you DEFINITELY need enzymes. There are enzymes that are specifically targeted to aid each organ and system of your body. Many argue that blood tests are better than urinalysis; I beg to differ. By the time something shows up in your blood it has already been in your body way too long. By conducting a urinalysis we can target the issue before it shows up in your labs. See TIPS #49, #54, #106, #142, #155, #160, #207, #219, #222, #276, #310, #320, and #346.

TIP #320:

There are two things I VERY RARELY miss and those are digestive enzymes at first bite of every meal and snack, and probiotics. This will definitely help your digestion and your intestinal flora. As your digestive system gets stronger, the afternoon drop will disappear and you will feel better and better as time goes by. You need a good quality digestive enzyme which will help you break down protein, carbs, gluten, fat. Or maybe you need a targeted one depending on what the issue is: Digestion, assimilation, diet, etc. See TIPS #49, #54, #106, #142, #155, #160, #207, #219, #222, #276, #310, #319, and #346.

TIP #321:

Pinch one nostril and breathe from the other one. Take 10 to 12 deep long inhalations and exhalations and then switch to the other nostril. This will oxygenate your brain and will help you feel more focused and less tired. See TIP #313.

TIP #322:

This is what I do to manage my time and make things easier for me during the week:

MONTHLY BASIS:

I buy enough beets, ginger, and turmeric. I disinfect them, peel them (except the beets), and cut them in 1" x 1" bite-size pieces. Wrap them with paper towels, cover them and keep them in the freezer. Use a separate container for each one. See TIPS #30, #31, and #41. I also buy enough frozen fruit (usually mixed berries) to last me a while avoiding the washing and disinfecting of fruit. The nutritional value of frozen fruit is not compromised.

WEEKLY BASIS:

In small containers or bags I add all the powders, seeds and nuts for the 6 days I am going to drink my smoothie. I usually do this on a weekend. See TIP #100.

In small bowls or bags I add the exact amount of combined fruit plus a 1" piece of beet, ginger, carrot, coconut, and turmeric. Fruit could be fresh and/or frozen, as I mentioned before. And I keep them in the freezer. See TIP #100.

I also try to buy pre-washed leafy green veggies to mix in with my smoothie when I am in a rush. Or disinfect and wash all of your greens at the same time and use your salad bag to keep them fresh longer. See TIP #136.

For all my supplements, I do the same: I have small bags and prepare them for a couple of weeks at a time.

TIP #323:

Airrosti is a localized fascia massage done by specialized chiropractors trained in this modality. It can expedite the healing process of several injuries and the sessions are targeted to the area.

TIP #324:

Recipes:	TIP#
Almond Milk	25
Body Scrub	330
Bone Health	28
Coconut Dessert	47
Coconut "Pudding"	91
Colds	74, 176
Facial Scrub	67
Facial Toner	356
Fruit Purée	288
Green Juice	12
Mouth Wash	60
Oatmeal	52, 130
Quinoa	88
Salad Dressing	124
Shea Butter	75
Smoothie	**100**
Sore Throats	74

Trail Mix	331
Vegetable Pico	304

TIP #325:

When you stink, you need zinc!!! If you have foul body odor, you need zinc. See TIP #363.

TIP #326:

Açai berries are low in sugar and are loaded with calcium and vitamin 'A'. See TIP #100.

TIP #327:

Traumeel is an excellent homeopathic ointment to aid with swelling and bruising. See TIP #332.

TIP #328:

Once in a while it is good to take the following to support the perfect function of your bladder: Cornsilk and hydrangea. If you have issues, always consult a physician first.

TIP #329:

Konjac noodles are a great source of fiber, hence very filling; they have no added preservatives, artificial colors or flavors. They come in all different shapes to make fettuccini, penne, orzo, angel hair, etc. They are already cooked; all you have to do is rinse them out and put them in a skillet to evaporate all the water in them. Proceed to add sauces, veggies, meat, etc. Great alternative as gluten-replacement products.

TIP #330:

Moisturizing body scrub:
1/2 cup of Coconut Oil
1 cup of Xylitol, Erythritol, or Stevia
10 drops Lavender Essential Oil (or your choice)

Combine all ingredients and store in a clean glass jar. Enjoy in your shower! See TIP #**299**.

TIP #331:

Trail Mix:
2 cups Pumpkin Seeds (unsalted)
1 1/2 cups Sunflower Seeds (unsalted)
1 cup Almonds (unsalted, coarsely chopped)
1/2 cup Medjool Dates (pitted and chopped)
2 cups Apple Rings (dried and unsweetened)
1 cup Coconut Flakes (organic and unsweetened)
1/3 cup Coconut Crystals

In a skillet heat coconut crystals on low, until melted.
Mix immediately with coconut flakes.
Wait until it cools down and crush it into small pieces.
Chop the apples.
Mix all ingredients and enjoy!

TIP #332:

There are several products I use for inflammation (internal and external) and for bruising:
Arnica: I brew it and take it as tea. You can also find it in the form of an ointment and you can rub it on the bruised area.
Turmeric: Used in a therapeutic dose. A good reliable brand I have used is Terry's Naturals. See TIP #327.

TIP #333:

Yerbabuena (known as spearmint) tea is very good when you feel nauseous. Just boil 3 to 4 leaves in hot water for 5 minutes. Take the leaves out and sweeten it with raw honey (if unable to drink by itself).

TIP #334:

Cupping is an ancient treatment which has existed since 300 to 400 BC. Suction cups of different sizes are applied to the skin to improve circulation through the tissues which can actually help heal faster. It was widely used by Michael Phelps in the Olympics of 2016.

TIP #335:

Do you feel exhausted? Does it take all the energy in the world to get out of bed? Do you have to pull over when you are driving because you are tired? How long can you go without eating between meals? Do you need caffeine and, if so, how late do you need to drink it to keep going? Do your sugars drop at night? Anxiety or depression? Night sweats? Nightmares? You might be suffering from Adrenal Fatigue. If you do, the following get depleted very fast: B-5, B-6, C, calcium, magnesium, potassium, and zinc. Seek help. There are different things that can support your adrenals: Ashwaganda, enzymes, pantothenic acid (B-5).

TIP #336:

You can disinfect your veggies and fruit with vinegar and water or with Rebel Green Veggie Clean. See TIPS #100 #208, and #299.

TIP #337:

Collagen is the most abundant protein in the body; it stimulates collagen production in the body aiding joints, bones, and skin.   I love Pure Marine Collagen Peptides.

TIP #338:

It is important to pay attention to your eating habits. We need to let our digestive system rest. So it is good to let 5 to 6 hours go by between meals. This will really help your endocrine system. I let 12 hours go by between my last bite of the day and the first of the morning. Nowadays people call it intermittent fasting.

TIP #339:

If you happen to have a live mosquito trapped in your ear, put a sliced sweet fruit next to your ear to see if it finds its way out. Seek professional help, otherwise.

TIP #340:

If you crave carbohydrates, try using chlorella tablets which help detoxify. If they don't work, try specific enzymes to digest them. See TIP #219.

TIP #341:

Marshmallow balances excessive secretions. It needs to be taken on an empty stomach.

TIP #342:

In order to have a healthier thyroid, you might try the following:
Don't drink tap water. Tap water is loaded with chlorine which absorbs iodine.
Stop eating anything that contains barley, rye, and wheat which is in almost all breads; these can cause inflammation. Stay away from hydrogenated oils and preservatives. See TIPS #92, #187, #193, #249, #257, #281, #345, and #352.

TIP #343:

Capsicum is great for cuts which bleed excessively; it is also known to be used sublingual for heart attacks. Please call an Ambulance before you administer it.

TIP #344:

Biotin, yellow dock, horsetail, garlic, and Omega 3's are great for hair and nails.

TIP #345:

HYPO-THYROID:

Absolutely get away from gluten, sugar, corn, citrus, refined grains, dairy, and soy. See TIPS #92, #187, #193, #249, #257, #281, #342, and #352.

TIP #346:

Do you want to experience better digestion and elimination?

Chew, chew, and chew each bite 20 to 30 times.
Eat plenty of fiber in the form of fresh fruit and veggies.
Drink plenty of water (See TIP #200).
Eat probiotic foods or pills every day (See TIP #142).
Take a general digestive enzymes with every meal and
snack, especially if the food is cooked. See TIPS #54,
#106, #142, #160, #207, #319, and #320.
Avoid sugar, alcohol, caffeine, and processed foods.
Eat sunflower seeds, hemp seeds, pumpkin seeds, chia
seeds or flaxseeds every day.

TIP #347:

Leaky Gut?
Repair it using supplements and foods: aloe vera gel,
cabbage juice, digestive enzymes, and most importantly,
consult an alternative doctor.

TIP #348:

The difference between an infusion and a decoction is the
method of preparation. An infusion is when you let an herb
stand in water overnight. A decoction is when you boil the
herb.

TIP #349:

What do you consider "normal stool elimination?" We all
should go, at least, two to three times a day; **ideally every
time after a major meal**. This is considered optimal. Bristol
Stool has a scale that will aid us to understand how healthy
our elimination system is (which is part of digestion). There
are 7 different types of stool formation:

Type I: "Separate hard lumps, like nuts (hard to pass)", similar to rabbit pellets.

Type II: "Sausage-shaped but lumpy. This is the most destructive because of the size." This means you have had this stool sitting in your colon for several weeks.

Type III: "Like a sausage but with cracks on its surface."

TYPE IV: "Like a sausage or snake, smooth and soft."

TYPE V: "Soft blobs with clear-cut edges (passed easily)."

TYPE VI: "Fluffy pieces with ragged edges, a mushy stool."

TYPE VII: "Watery, no solid pieces. Entirely liquid."

Types I and II are severe constipation.
Types III and IV are considered normal.
Type V means you are probably lacking fiber.
Type VI and VII are diarrhea.

TIP #350:

There is a belief roaming around which sustains that arthritis sufferers should not eat night shades. Again, we are all not made the same. Try the following:
Right before summer get off night shades (bell peppers, eggplant, tomatoes, tomatillos, goji berries, carrots, regular potatoes, etc.) and then go crazy on tomatoes. See if this exacerbates the arthritis.

TIP #351:

Sulphur, in a powder form, is great to help acne and boils. Ingested it helps with eczema, collagen production, depression, psoriasis, and fibromyalgia. Check out the homeopathic products from Boiron.

TIP #352:

Iodine should not be taken across the board. There are different types for different organs:
Iodine with Potassium supports the thyroid
Iodine Elemental supports all other organs. See TIPS #92, #187, #193, #249, #257, #281, #342, and #345.

TIP #353:

When it comes to PREVENTING cancer, there are different ways of seeing it. If you take a wholistic point of view, we need not only consider the physical body, but also the emotional status and your diet.
1. We need to support our immune system by feeding it REAL food, food produced by Mother Earth. We need to eat things such as FRESH vegetables and fruits. If we are having a fruit cocktail, we buy fresh fruit and mix it and we do not eat it from a can. Canned fruit is NOT REAL food. STOP eating anything that is canned, bottled, processed, fried, or soaked in sauces which are loaded with sugar.
2. STOP eating SUGAR and its derivatives. See TIP#35.
3. STOP eating bread, tortillas, chips, etc. See TIP #286.
4. Eat fresh pasture-raised organic meats and wild-caught fish if you absolutely have to have meat.
5. Take digestive enzymes with every meal and snack. See TIP #106.
6. Take probiotics with every meal.
7. We need to check our stool. Do we poop every day, how often, what is the consistency of our excrement, etc. (See TIP #349 for more information on this subject.)
8. Are you constantly in a state of stress which is undermining your immune system? You need to find

balance in your life. You will not take anything with you when you are gone. There has to be a balance between work, family, fun, and time for yourself.

9. Emotions play a very important role in life. If you constantly entertain anger, jealousy, envy, unforgiveness, regret, etc., all these emotions play havoc inside of you too. Deal with them. Confront your stuff!!!! Live in peace. See TIP #378.

10. Drink water and nothing else (and not directly from a faucet unless you have a filtered system.)

11. And, of course, medicine - both allopathic and homeopathic - get help there too!!! It is a combination of all of the above. Humans are not made of parts, we are a WHOLE. *__Remember: Our body is our temple; it is our only expression in this physical experience. A very complex machine which will react to love and care. Stop treating it with violence. At the very end: You are what you eat, what you cannot eliminate, the emotions you cannot digest, and the stress YOU HAVE elected to experience in your life.__*

TIP #354:

Candida is a fungus which lives in small amounts in different parts of our body, but mainly in our gut. When we take too many antibiotics, eat too many refined sweets (sugar, refined flours, and starches), drink alcohol, have diabetes, or experience high levels of stress, we can experience a candida overgrowth. Do you experience itchy skin, eczema, vaginal burning, brain fog, lethargy, dry skin, fatigue, mood disorders? Your gut bacteria could be totally off. You can start balancing your gut flora by doing this for, at least, one month (check with your physician first.)

- Stop eating all sweets: bad and good, white flour, crackers, chips, all fruits (except berries - but keep them to a minimum), potatoes, corn, fried food, bottled juices and

drinks, anything packaged that contains sugar, potatoes or corn. (See TIP #35).
- Eat only green vegetables, leafy greens, and cauliflower.
- Eat organic pasture-raised white and red meat (no organ meat), and poultry or wild-caught fish. All broiled or grilled. No sauces.
- No dairy, except organic pasture-raised eggs.
- No alcoholic beverages, sodas, hi-energy drinks, sweeteners, flavor-added packages, or caffeine. Just water.
- Take a probiotic: 3 in the morning, 3 in the afternoon, and 3 in the evening away from food for 2 weeks. For the following 2 weeks take 2 in the morning, 2 in the afternoon, and 2 in the evening away from food. Try to get a good source of probiotic; at the end cheap turns out to be expensive.
- Take 2 capsules of a general digestive enzyme with every meal and snack. See TIPS #106 and #319.
- Buy black walnut and olive leaf in liquid form and take it twice a day, morning and evening, away from food.

By doing this, you will be starving the fungus and you might experience skin eruptions and other yeast symptoms. You might have to repeat this cycle two or three times.

After your symptoms have cleared up, you can take 2 probiotics with a meal every day and continue taking the digestive enzymes with every meal and snack.

Introduce one item at a time into your diet and wait 4 to 5 days to see if your body reacts to it. If symptoms persist, consult a physician.

TIP #355:

Children with seizures? Investigate the keto diet. There are a myriad of studies supporting that the brain needs fat to survive and it has helped many kids.

TIP #356:

As a natural facial toner for my face:
Boil enough water for 1/2 cup; turn the burner off.
Steep a teabag of chamomile (manzanilla) for about 30
minutes. Take the teabag out and let it cool down.
Once it is at room temperature pour into your bottle and
use all over your face, neck, and body. I leave it in the
refrigerator. It is very refreshing and hydrating.

TIP #357:

Kids with ADHD? Research the Feingold Program. It is an elimination system which basically avoids anything with petroleum-based products such as artificial flavorings and fragrances and the majority of dyes. It takes parents and children through an eye-opening tour of food.

TIP #358:

Facial Flex is a device I use for facial exercises which was initially invented for patients who had suffered a stroke. It helps tighten your jawline and neck.

TIP #359:

Healthy For Good is a fantastic movement which encourages you to eat smart, move more, and be well. Check them out.

TIP #360:

What helps me soothe the itchiness from mosquito bites is honey, apple cider vinegar, aloe vera, and colloidal silver.

Just rub any of these products on the bite. See TIPS #121, #227, #255, and #367.

TIP #361:

Support your liver with herbs such as dandelion, milk thistle, and burdock. Eat foods which are rich in sulphur: Garlic, onion, and cabbage.

TIP #362:

Goji berries are a great antioxidant superfood. I add it to my smoothie. See TIP #100.

TIP #363:

Soak in the tub with 1/2 cup of baking soda to eliminate strong body odor. See TIP # 325.

TIP #364:

Make your own cereal:
Steel cut oatmeal, chopped apples, chopped dates, chopped almonds, a bit of maple syrup and cashew milk.

TIP #365:

We should ban Children's Menus in all restaurants. They all contain highly processed, sugar-loaded and fried food; nothing that is actually nourishing our kids. And then we wonder why adult-related diseases are presenting themselves in kids?? Really!!!! French fries, sliders, Mac and cheese, pizza, ice-cream, chicken

fingers (breaded), pancakes with powdered sugar, sodas, bottled apple juice, etc. etc. etc. It is absolutely ludicrous. Do you need ideas? See TIP #366.

TIP #366:

Let's feed our children cut fruit in the shape of a fish, a piece of meat on top of mashed potatoes shaped as a boat, veggies with grilled chicken, freshly squeezed orange juice, water, carbonated water with a wedge of lime, lemon, grapefruit, orange, etc, and sweetened with stevia or maple syrup or raw honey, scrambled eggs in the form of a UFO, unsweetened shredded coconut with nuts and maple syrup, potato and kale in the shape of stars.   See TIP #365.

TIP #367:

To avoid getting bit by mosquitoes rub basil on yourself or boil basil and pour the tea in a bottle and constantly spray it on you while you are outside. See TIPS #121, #227, #255, and #360.

TIP #368:

TIPS #162 through #173 and #183 through #194 stress the importance of a **WIDE** variety of foods. We, humans, tend to get too comfortable eating the same food over and over again depleting our bodies from **ALL** the vitamins and minerals.

TIP #369:

If your pH is below 6.5 you are too ***ACIDIC.***

Eat these alkaline foods:
Almonds, apples, asparagus, avocados, bananas, broccoli, canteloupe, carrots, cherries, dates, figs, garlic, grapefruit, grapes, kiwis, lemons, limes, mushrooms, onions, oranges, papaya, parsley, peaches, pears, pineapple, quinoa, spinach, tomatoes, watermelon, wild rice.

Remember all your vegetables and fruits need to be organic. See TIP #20 and #21.

TIP #370:

If your pH is above 7 you are too ***ALKALINE.***

Eat these acidic foods:
Beef (organic and pasture raised), blackberries, blueberries, brown rice, butter, cashews, chicken (pasture raised and organic), cranberries, eggs (pasture raised), fish (wild-caught), black beans, kidney beans, lima beans, navy beans, pinto beans, raspberries, oats, pecans, plums, pumpkin seeds, soy milk (100% certified organic), strawberries, sunflower seeds, turkey (organic) walnuts.

Remember all your vegetables and fruits need to be organic. See TIP #20 and #21.

TIP #371:

Rubbing alcohol is not good for you. It is unsafe to drink it because it has a combination of the alcohol plus bitter poisons which make it toxic. My question to you is: Doesn't the skin absorb everything you rub on to it? I use it when strictly necessary. My preference is witch hazel.

TIP #372:

Eggs, as long as they are pasture-raised and organic, are good for you. It is a complete food. When you start tampering with Mother Nature and start eating whites, or liquid whites, or powdered eggs, etc. that is when it becomes a problem; those are not eggs, they are PROCESSED FOOD and it is not good for you. Eggs are a wholesome food.

TIP #373:

Cilantro is an excellent herb to use for metal detoxification. Chop it up and sprinkle it over eggs, rice, quinoa, etc.

TIP #374:

Once or twice a year I have a foot detox bath to draw some of the metal accumulation we have due to mere modern living. You can find these devices on the internet; I enjoy the EB Pro Energy Balancing System. You just need to follow the instructions precisely and drink lots of water throughout the day so you don't get dehydrated. Or go to a chiropractor who provides this service.

TIP #375:

In order to blend my smoothie, I need a professional blender. The only brands I trust to disintegrate all that I put in my smoothie is VitaMix and BlendTec. See TIP #100.

TIP #376:

I make "Happy Water" which is a mix of different Bach Flowers to balance your emotions. Try it out. Make your own mix depending on how you feel; add 10 drops to a glass of water and drink it in the morning when you wake up.

TIP #377:

It is as important to drink enough water as it is to over drink. The water companies have made us all believe that we need to intake endless amounts of water and this is not true. If we take too much water we can deplete our bodies from precious minerals. See TIPS #3, #4, and #200 (to calculate how much water you should take.)

TIP #378:

Issues hanging on to things? Unresolved feelings? Resentments? Grief? Anger? Here are some exercises which helped me tremendously:
- Grab a pillow and talk to it while you are hitting it. Do it for several minutes until your emotions start showing up and continue until you feel more at ease.
- Write a letter to whomever you resent: Mom, dad, spouse, sibling, boss, etc. Pour your heart out. Then read the letter OUT LOUD several times. When you feel you have expressed all you need to and emotions don't flare anymore, burn it: forever GONE!!
- Seek an emotional release specialist to aid you in dealing with this: Psychology, Reiki, Emotional Healing, Hypnosis, etc.; choose whichever technique suits you but do work through them. Ignoring them will not make them disappear and will not allow you to evolve, emotionally speaking.

TIP #379:

Issues with emotions? One of the best books which was recommended to me by a very dear friend and holistic doctor based in Los Angeles, CA is called "The Telomere Effect". It is a fantastic way to detach your feelings from your actions and being able to process them in a different way. It entails referring to yourself in the third person. Try it!

TIP #380:

Aloe vera juice is excellent for digestion and it improves absorption of nutrients. I drink one tablespoon daily for about a month and I do this once a year.

TIP #381:

We need to learn to disconnect from our daily routine and stress. It only takes 5 minutes if you totally shift your gear to something unrelated so you can de-stress. This is called recovery time. It is very different from resting time. Restful time is when you are physically resting but your mind is focused on how to solve "x" or "y" problems. Recovery time is when you shift your focus for 5 minutes or 1 hour (time is irrelevant) and do something totally unrelated (Harvard University).

TIP #382:

If you are battling with strep throat or sore throat, this can help get rid of it:
Mix apple cider vinegar with the "mother" and water and gargle throughout the day.

Mix the same amount of cayenne pepper and raw organic honey and dab with a cotton swab in the back of the throat. You can also take one teaspoon of this mixture once a day.

TIP #383:

Try to do your daily routines with a different hand to make new brain connections: Brush your teeth with your opposite hand; when you eat use the opposite hand as well, etc. This will stimulate your brain and make it healthier and agile.

TIP #384:

EVENING ROUTINE:

I take two different enzymes to support the liver and another one to support the circulatory system. And I also take an enzyme to aid sleeping too. I also do a short session of heart math or EFT to clear my emotions.

TIP #385:

Achy body: Take a bath in Epsom salts to relax your muscles.

TIP #386:

If you need throat lozenges when you have a cold or a sore throat, I would highly recommend the brand Zarbee's. They are made of natural ingredients with no refined sugar or artificial flavors. They come from Canada.

TIP #387:

IN A NUT SHELL:

NO to canned and bottled sauces or salsas.
NO to colorings or dyes, et al: Red, Yellow, Violet, Blue, etc. regardless of the number that follows.
NO to chips of any sort.
NO to plastic containers unless you only use them to store cold or frozen items.
NO to white flour: Bread, flour tortillas, pancakes, rice, crackers, etc.
NO to processed sugar : candy, ice cream, sweets, etc. (remember sugar comes under many different names: sucrose, dextrose, fructose, corn syrup, etc.)
NO to animal milk (unless it is organic and pasture-raised with no other added or deducted ingredients and only if you cannot live without it.)
NO to egg whites and egg beaters.
NO to processed cheese.
NO to tephlon.
NO consuming of Dirty Dozen if they are not organic.
NO to soya.
NO to pumping iron or crazy machinery.
YES to homemade fresh salsas.
YES to all fruits and vegetables.
YES to organic pasture-raised meats. (if you have to eat them.)
YES to wild caught fish (if you choose to incorporate it in your diet.)
YES to glass containers.
YES to cooking with stainless steels pots and pans.
YES to 50% of your diet being raw.
YES to exercise (15 minutes daily minimum).
YES to recovery time during the day.
YES to continuous natural movement.
YES to reading the ingredients and not only the front of the package (regardless of what the front label says.)

YES to nut based milks as long as you read the ingredients and they don't contain sucrose, dextrose, carragenan, and natural flavors.
YES to pasture-raised eggs.
YES to 100% certified organic soya.
YES to nuts and grains such as quinoa, buckwheat, job's tears.
YES to all spices and herbs.
YES to Clean 15.
YES to sleeping a minimum of 6 hours.

YES, IT IS EXPENSIVE; but it is your health. Would you put it on the line?

YES TO A PAIN-FREE LIFE!!!

GLOSSARY:

RESOURCES

Aloe Life
Annie's Heirloom Seeds
Applied Environmental Microbiology
Bedford Hospital (UK Scientists)
BodyBio
Cambridge University Hospital
Dr. Anstett, Thomas
Dr. Christianson
Dr. Fritchey, Philip
Dr. Muñoz, Luis
Dr. Newkirk, Elaine
Dr. Shumway, Marcus
Dulce Revolución
EB Pro Energy Balancing System
EFT (Emotional Freedom Technique)
Egoscue (Peter Egoscue)
Environmental Working Group (EWG)
Fit Brain
Food Matters
Food Revolution
Frontier Coop
Geopharm
Go Raw
Harvard Health Education
Harvard Medical School
Hay House
Heart Math
High Mowing Seeds
His Good Herbs
Know Cow
José Pamies
Journal of American Science 2011
Journal of Glaucoma 2016
Kinesio Taping
Leo Hart

Local Harvest
Lumosity
National Center on Health, Physical Activity and Disability (NCHPAD)
National Library of Medicine
National Research Council
Natural Society
Ocean Robbins
Organic Gardening
Pure Healing Foods
Robert Holden
Seeds of Change
Sun Warrior
Super Foods for Super Health
Teresa Tapp
The Tapping Solution
University of Washington (Prof. Steinemman)